CARDIOLOGY RESEARCH AND CLINICAL DEVELOPMENTS

PULMONARY HYPERTENSION

PATHOGENESIS, DIAGNOSIS, AND TREATMENTS

CARDIOLOGY RESEARCH AND CLINICAL DEVELOPMENTS

Additional books in this series can be found on Nova's website under the Series tab.

Additional e-books in this series can be found on Nova's website under the e-books tab.

CARDIOLOGY RESEARCH AND CLINICAL DEVELOPMENTS

PULMONARY HYPERTENSION

PATHOGENESIS, DIAGNOSIS, AND TREATMENTS

HUILI GAN
EDITOR

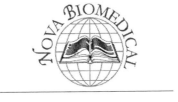

Nova Science Publishers, Inc.
New York

Copyright © 2012 by Nova Science Publishers, Inc.

All rights reserved. No part of this book may be reproduced, stored in a retrieval system or transmitted in any form or by any means: electronic, electrostatic, magnetic, tape, mechanical photocopying, recording or otherwise without the written permission of the Publisher.

For permission to use material from this book please contact us:
Telephone 631-231-7269; Fax 631-231-8175
Web Site: http://www.novapublishers.com

NOTICE TO THE READER

The Publisher has taken reasonable care in the preparation of this book, but makes no expressed or implied warranty of any kind and assumes no responsibility for any errors or omissions. No liability is assumed for incidental or consequential damages in connection with or arising out of information contained in this book. The Publisher shall not be liable for any special, consequential, or exemplary damages resulting, in whole or in part, from the readers' use of, or reliance upon, this material. Any parts of this book based on government reports are so indicated and copyright is claimed for those parts to the extent applicable to compilations of such works.

Independent verification should be sought for any data, advice or recommendations contained in this book. In addition, no responsibility is assumed by the publisher for any injury and/or damage to persons or property arising from any methods, products, instructions, ideas or otherwise contained in this publication.

This publication is designed to provide accurate and authoritative information with regard to the subject matter covered herein. It is sold with the clear understanding that the Publisher is not engaged in rendering legal or any other professional services. If legal or any other expert assistance is required, the services of a competent person should be sought. FROM A DECLARATION OF PARTICIPANTS JOINTLY ADOPTED BY A COMMITTEE OF THE AMERICAN BAR ASSOCIATION AND A COMMITTEE OF PUBLISHERS.

Additional color graphics may be available in the e-book version of this book.

Library of Congress Cataloging-in-Publication Data

Pulmonary hypertension : pathogenesis, diagnosis, and treatments / editor, Huili Gan.
 p. ; cm.
 Includes bibliographical references and index.
 ISBN 978-1-61470-556-7 (hardcover)
 1.Pulmonary hypertension. I. Gan, Huili.
 [DNLM: 1. Hypertension, Pulmonary. WG 340]
 RC776.P87P85652 2011
 616.2'4--dc23

2011024537

Published by Nova Science Publishers, Inc. † New York

Contents

Preface		vii
Editor's Affiliation		xi
Chapter I	Pulmonary Hypertension: Pathogenesis, Diagnosis, and Treatments *Jing-bin Huang and Jian Liang*	1
Chapter II	Possible Bridging to Final Repair in Eisenmenger Syndrome *Ming-Tai Lin and Yih-Sharng Chen*	57
Chapter III	The Management of Congenital Systemic-to-pulmonary Shunt and Advanced Pulmonary Artery Hypertension *Hui-Li Gan and Jian-Qun Zhang*	79
Chapter IV	Systemic Inflammatory Response Syndrome Associated with Pulmonary Endarterectomy in Patients with Chronic Thromboembolic Pulmonary Hypertension *Pavel Maruna, Andrew A. Klein, Jan Kunstyr, Katerina M. Plocova, Frantisek Mlejnsky, David Ambroz, and Jaroslav Lindner*	101

Chapter V	Liver Transplantation and Pulmonary Hypertension *Michael Ramsay*	**117**
Chapter VI	Pulmonary Hypertension in the Down Syndrome Population *Clifford L. Cua, Louis G. Chicoine,* *Leif D. Nelin, and Mary Mullen*	**137**
Index		**147**

Preface

Pulmonary hypertension is a complex disease that causes significant morbidity and mortality and is clinically characterized by an increase in pulmonary vascular resistance. The histopathology is marked by vascular proliferation/fibrosis, remodeling, and vessel obstruction. In this book, the authors present current research in the study of the pathogenesis, diagnosis and treatment of pulmonary hypertension. Topics discussed include the pathophysiology of Eisenmenger Syndrome (ES) and an evaluation of differences between ES and pulmonary arterial hypertension; pulmonary endarterectomy as an effective treatment for chronic thromboembolic pulmonary hypertension; liver transplantation and pulmonary hypertension and the possible etiologies of pulmonary hypertension in Down Syndrome children.

Chapter I - Pulmonary hypertension (PH) is a complex disease that causes significant morbidity and mortality and is clinically characterized by an increase in pulmonary vascular resistance. The histopathology is marked by vascular proliferation/fibrosis, remodeling, and vessel obstruction. Development of pulmonary hypertension involves the complex interaction of multiple vascular effectors at all anatomic levels of the arterial wall. Subsequent vasoconstriction, thrombosis, and inflammation ensue, leading to vessel wall remodeling and cellular hyperproliferation as the hallmarks of severe disease. Recent studies have provided a glimpse at certain molecular pathways that contribute to pathogenesis; these have led to the identification of attractive targets for therapeutic intervention. The current conceptual framework should allow for future studies to refine our understanding of the molecular pathogenesis of pulmonary hypertension and improve the therapeutic regimen for this disease. The treatment of pulmonary hypertensionhas evolved considerably over the past few years as the number of therapeutic options available to treat this disease has increased. In this Review we attempt to summarize the current knowledge of the pathogenesis of pulmonary hypertension, in relation to the therapies presently available and those that could become available in the near future. The use of prostacyclin and its analogs, calcium-channel blockers, endothelin-receptor antagonists and phosphordiesterase type 5 inhibitors is reviewed. Newer concepts, such as the use of combination therapy, and the potential for long-term disease amelioration and improvement of outcomes, are also discussed. In addition, we review the novel emerging therapies, such as imatinib, fasudil, simvastatin, ghrelin and vasoactive intestinal peptide, which hold therapeutic potential for disease modification as well as treatment of symptoms.

Chapter II - Congenital heart disease (CHD)-related pulmonary arterial hypertension (PAH) remains a major concern despite advances in cardiac surgery. The currently accepted mechanism of CHD-related PAH holds that increased pulmonary blood flow and pressure trigger unfavorable vascular remodeling. Eisenmenger syndrome (ES), the most advanced form, is defined as CHD with an initially large systemic-to-pulmonary shunt, that induces severe pulmonary vascular disease and PAH, with resultant reversal of the shunt and central cyanosis. Eisenmenger syndrome (ES) is usually considered inoperable, but recent success of advanced vasodilator therapies for idiopathic PAH has offered new hope for ES patients. This review initially provides an overview of the pathophysiology of ES and then an evaluation of differences between ES and other forms of PAH, including increased survival, more effective adaptation of RV, polyclonal endothelial cell proliferation, and less occurrence of mutations in the Type II bone morphogenetic protein receptor. Up to one third of ES patients demonstrated maintaining some degree of pulmonary vasoreactivity. With increased understanding of the mechanisms of developing ES, several targeted therapies for PAH associated with CHD, including endothelin receptor antagonists and phosphodiesterase Type-5 inhibitors, have been proved to be effective in reducing pulmonary vascular resistance and symptoms. Pairs of staged surgical approaches aimed to reverse vascular remodeling, such as pulmonary arterial band, one-way flap and Mustard operation, have also been attempted to limit flow and shear stress on pulmonary circulation. Some selected patients exhibited promising improvement in functional class and even achieved final total repair. In this paper, we review the small-scale advanced studies and classify them, in an anatomic manner, into pre-tricuspid, post-tricuspid and complex types of

CHD. Size of the defect, magnitude of the shunt, changes of vascular resistance, pulmonary pressure, saturation and exercise tolerance, and percentages of achievement of final repair are summarized and discussed. Further large-scale prospective investigations are required to elucidate both the benefits of these novel approaches in ES and the optimal time for initiating treatment.

Chapter III - Our objective was to investigate the relationship between the long-term survival of surgical treatment and preoperative pulmonary vascular resistance (PVR) and pulmonary to systemic flow ratio (Qp/Qs) in congenital systemic-to-pulmonary shunt with andadvanced pulmonary hypertension.

Chapter IV - Pulmonary endarterectomy (PEA) is an effective treatment for chronic thromboembolic pulmonary hypertension (CTEPH). There are recent experimental findings suggesting the involvement of circulating cytokines such as interleukin-6 (IL-6), IL-8 and tumor necrosis factor-α (TNFα) in hemodynamic instability in the perioperative course of PEA. In a prospective study, the authors tested the hypothesis that elevated acute-phase reactants, induced by uncomplicated PEA, may influence haemodynamic parameters after PEA.

Chapter V - Portopulmonary hypertension is found in 5-6% of patients with portal hypertension. This may or may not be associated with liver cirrhosis. If cirrhosis is present the severity of the liver cirrhosis does not correlate with the degree of pulmonary hypertension. The diagnosis of portopulmonary hypertension includes a mean pulmonary artery pressure of greater than 25 mm Hg at rest and a pulmonary vascular resistance of greater than 240 dyncs.s.cm^{-5} and the presence of portal hypertension. Approximately 20% of patients with liver cirrhosis presenting for liver transplantation will have increased pulmonary artery pressures, but in the majority of patients this is the result of intravascular volume overload, together with a high flow state that is typically seen in patients with liver cirrhosis and this may be further affected by the presence of a cirrhotic cardiomyopathy. However the key differentiator of these causes of pulmonary hypertension from true portopulmonary hypertension is that in this group the pulmonary vascular resistance is normal or low. The etiology of portopulmonary hypertension is not well understood. Initially endothelial dysfunction in the pulmonary arterioles may occur as the result of sheer stress forces from the high velocity circulation and the toxic effects of inflammatory molecules that are either not cleared by the liver or are released by the diseased liver. The clinical symptoms may be minimal in the early phases of the disease but as it progresses shortness of breath, chest pain, fatigue, palpitations and syncope may present. However these symptoms are not distinct from those of progressive liver disease, therefore all liver transplant candidates should be screened for portopulmonary hypertension. The current screening tool is the transthoracic Doppler echocardiogram. If the right ventricular systolic pressure is 50 mm Hg. or greater a right heart catheterization should be performed and the pulmonary vascular resistance calculated. Once the diagnosis of portopulmonary hypertension has been made a careful assessment of right ventricular function is required by echocardiography. Liver transplantation will treat many of these patients but not all, and it cannot be predicted which patients will respond to transplantation. The risks of liver transplantation increase with the severity of the pulmonary hypertension and those patients with evidence of right heart dysfunction should undergo pulmonary vasodilator therapy prior to consideration for transplant.

Chapter VI - Down syndrome (DS) is a common genetic disorder with protean manifestations. Children with DS are at risk for multiple medical issues that are well described; however, a potentially underappreciated condition that appears to have a high prevalence in this patient population is pulmonary hypertension (PH). The increased prevalence of PH in this population may have serious short and long-term consequences. The causes of PH in the DS population are not precisely known, but may be due to multiple other associated medical conditions that these children have concurrently, or due to shared biological features. We review the literature that describes the possible etiologies of PH in DS children with the hope that further research is performed to better define this complicated population.

Editor's Affiliation

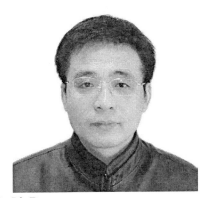

Hui-Li Gan, MD, Ph.D
Professor of Cardiac Surgery
Department of Cardiac Surgery,
Beijing Anzhen Hospital, Capital Medical University,
Beijing Institute of Heart, Lung and Blood Vessel Diseases,
Beijing 100029, China

Conflict of Interest Disclosures: The author (Hui-Li Gan) now serves as a local experienced surgeon in the phase III trials --the CHEST-1 and CHEST-2 study--on Riociguat, a novel drug that is currently in clinical development by Bayer Schering Pharma
Sources of Funding: This article was partially supported by a grant (#81070041) from National Nature Science Foundation of China to Dr. Gan.)

In: Pulmonary Hypertension
Editor: Huili Gan

ISBN: 978-1-61470-556-7
© 2012 Nova Science Publishers, Inc.

Chapter I

Pulmonary Hypertension: Pathogenesis, Diagnosis, and Treatments

Jing-bin Huang and Jian Liang
Department of Cardiothoracic Surgery, The Affiliated Ruikang Hospital
of Guangxi Traditional Chinese Medical College, 10 Huadong Road,
Nanning, Guangxi Zhuang Autonomous Region, China

Abstract

Pulmonary hypertension (PH) is a complex disease that causes significant morbidity and mortality and is clinically characterized by an increase in pulmonary vascular resistance. The histopathology is marked by vascular proliferation/fibrosis, remodeling, and vessel obstruction. Development of pulmonary hypertension involves the complex interaction of multiple vascular effectors at all anatomic levels of the arterial wall. Subsequent vasoconstriction, thrombosis, and inflammation ensue, leading to vessel wall remodeling and cellular hyperproliferation as the hallmarks of severe disease. Recent studies have provided a glimpse at certain molecular pathways that contribute to pathogenesis; these have led to the identification of attractive targets for therapeutic intervention. The current conceptual framework should allow for future studies to refine our understanding of the molecular pathogenesis of pulmonary hypertension and improve the therapeutic regimen for this disease. The treatment of pulmonary hypertensionhas evolved considerably over the past few years as the number of therapeutic options available to treat this disease has increased. In this Review we attempt to summarize the current knowledge of the pathogenesis of pulmonary hypertension, in relation to the therapies presently available and those that could become available in the near future. The use of prostacyclin and its analogs, calcium-channel blockers, endothelin-receptor antagonists and phosphordiesterase type 5 inhibitors is reviewed. Newer concepts, such as the use of combination therapy, and the potential for long-term disease amelioration and improvement of outcomes, are also discussed. In addition, we review the novel emerging therapies, such as imatinib, fasudil, simvastatin, ghrelin and vasoactive intestinal peptide, which hold therapeutic potential for disease modification as well as treatment of symptoms.

Keywords: endothelin-receptor antagonists, phosphodiesterase type 5 inhibitors, prostacyclin, pulmonary hypertension

Introduction

Pulmonary hypertension (PH) is a complex disease that causes significant morbidity and mortality and is clinically characterized by an increase in pulmonary vascular resistance. The histopathology is marked by vascular proliferation/fibrosis, remodeling, and vessel obstruction. PHis defined as a mean pulmonary artery pressure (PAP) of greater than 25 mmHg at rest or at least 30 mmHg during exercise. These rises in PAP have to be associated with elevated pulmonary vascular resistance (PVR), and a mean pulmonary wedge pressure and left ventricular end diastolic pressure of less than 15 mmHg for diagnosis of PH.It should be noted that PH is not a disease but a pathophysiological parameter: a pulmonary arterial blood pressure exceeding the upper limits of normalcy. [1] PH occurs in a variety of clinical situations and is associated with a spectrum of histological patterns of abnormalities.PH is a common denominator of a heterogeneous group of disorders that differ in risk factor profile, eliciting factors, histopathological appearance, response to various therapies and prognosis.

In 1957, PH was already divided into 5 classes based on the underlying cause: chronic bronchitis and emphysema, left to right shunt, primary pulmonary hypertension, primary pulmonary arteriosclerosis and pulmonary embolism. [2] Advances in histopathology and understanding of disease pathogenesis resulted in renewed classifications in 1973 and 1998. In 1998, the WHO (Evian) classification system was proposed, which sought to categorize different forms of PH according to similarities in pathophysiological mechanisms, clinical presentation and therapeutic options.[3] In 2003 in Venice, modifications were made to this system, with the aim of making it more comprehensive, easier to follow and more practical for clinicians.[4] Underlining the impact of the development of various treatment modalities in recent years, the latest WHO classification (2008, Dana Point, CA, USA) was proposed (Table 1).

Table 1. Clinical classification of pulmonary hypertensionestablished in Venice, Italy, in 2003, and the current classification, established in Dana Point, CA, USA, in 2008

Venice, 2003	Dana Point, 2008
1. Pulmonary hypertension	1. Pulmonary hypertension
1.1. Idiopathic	1.1. Idiopathic
1.2. Familial	1.2. Heritable
1.3. Associated with:	1.2.1. BMPR2
1.3.1. Collagen vascular diseases	1.2.2. ALK-1, endoglin (with or without hereditary hemorrhagic telangiectasia)
1.3.2. Congenital systemic-pulmonary shunts	1.2.3. Unknown
1.3.3. Portal hypertension	1.3. Drug- and toxin-induced
1.3.4. Infection with the human immunodeficiency virus	1.4. Associated with
1.3.5. Drugs/toxins	1.4.1. Connective tissue diseases
1.3.6. Others (thyroid diseases, hereditary hemorrhagic telangiectasia, hemoglobinopathies, Gaucher's disease, myeloproliferative disorders, and splenectomy)	1.4.2. Human immunodeficiency virus infection
1.4. Associated with significant capillary or venous involvement	1.4.3. Portal hypertension
1.4.1. Pulmonary veno-occlusive disease	1.4.4. Congenital heart diseases
1.4.2. Pulmonary capillary hemangiomatosis	1.4.5. Schistosomiasis

Table 1. (Continued)

Venice, 2003	Dana Point, 2008
1.5. Persistent PH of the newborn	1.4.6. Chronic hemolytic anemia
	1.5. Persistent pulmonary hypertensionof the newborn
	1'. Pulmonary veno-occlusive disease and/or pulmonary capillary hemangiomatosis
2. Pulmonary venous hypertension	2. pulmonary hypertension owing to left heart disease
2.1. Left ventricular or left atrial heart disease	2.1. Systolic dysfunction
2.2. Left valvular heart disease	2.2. Diastolic dysfunction
	2.3. Valvular disease
3. Pulmonary hypertension associated with lung disease, hypoxemia, or both	3. Pulmonary hypertension owing to lung diseases and/or hypoxia
3.1. COPD	3.1. COPD
3.2. Interstitial lung disease	3.2. Interstitial lung disease
3.3. Sleep-disordered breathing	3.3. Other lung diseases with mixed restrictive and obstructive pattern
3.4. Alveolar hypoventilation	3.4. Sleep-disordered breathing
3.5. Chronic exposure to high altitudes	3.5. Alveolar hypoventilation disorders
3.6. Developmental abnormalities	3.6. Chronic exposure to high altitude
	3.7. Developmental abnormalities
4. Pulmonary hypertension due to embolic disease, chronic thrombotic disease, or both	4. Chronic thromboembolic pulmonary hypertension
4.1. Thromboembolic obstruction of proximal pulmonary arteries	
4.2. Obstruction of distal pulmonary arteries	
4.3. Nonthrombotic pulmonary embolism (tumor, parasites, foreign body)	
5. Miscellaneous	5. Pulmonary hypertension with unclear multifactorial mechanisms

Venice, 2003	Dana Point, 2008
Sarcoidosis, histiocytosis X, lymphangioleiomyomatosis, compression of pulmonary vessels (adenopathy, tumor, and fibrosing mediastinitis)	5.1. Hematologic disorders: myeloproliferative disorders, splenectomy 5.2. Systemic disorders: sarcoidosis, pulmonary Langerhans cell histiocytosis: lymphangioleiomyomatosis, neurofibromatosis, vasculitis 5.3. Metabolic disorders: glycogen storage disease, Gaucher disease, thyroid disorders 5.4. Others: tumoral obstruction, fibrosing mediastinitis, chronic renal failure on dialysis

BMPR2: bone morphogenetic protein receptor, type 2; and ALK-1: activin receptor-like kinase-1.Adapted from Simonneau et al. [5]

Pathogenic Mechanisms

The pathogenesis of PH involves three major processes that contribute to narrowing of the pulmonary artery. The first, vasoconstriction, occurs as a result of an imbalance between vasodilators and vasoconstrictors in the pulmonary circulation. Vascular smooth muscle and endothelial cell proliferation result in vascular remodeling. Finally, coagulation abnormalities result in thrombosis *in situ*, which contributes to elevated PVR.

The histopathology is marked by vascular proliferation/fibrosis, remodeling, and vessel obstruction. Development of PH involves the complex interaction of multiple vascular effectors at all anatomic levels of the arterial wall. Subsequent vasoconstriction, thrombosis, and inflammation ensue, leading to vessel wall remodeling and cellular hyperproliferation as the hallmarks of severe disease. These processes are influenced by genetic predisposition as well as diverse endogenous and exogenous stimuli.

It has become increasingly clear that development of PH entails a complex, multifactorial pathophysiology. Although genetic mutations, exogenous exposures, and acquired disease states can predispose to PH, no one factor identified thus far is sufficient alone to drive fully the pathogenic process. Similar to carcinogenesis in which a susceptible person with a specific genetic mutation requires additional injuries to manifest disease, a "multiple-hit" hypothesis has emerged to explain the progression to clinical PH (Figure1).

Cellular Mechanisms

Pulmonary hypertension has a multifactorial pathobiology. Vasoconstriction, remodeling of the pulmonary vessel wall, and thrombosis contribute to increased pulmonary vascular resistance in PH. The process of pulmonary vascular remodeling involves all layers of the vessel wall and is complicated by cellular heterogeneity within each compartment of the pulmonary arterial wall. Indeed, each cell type (endothelial, smooth muscle, and fibroblast), as well as inflammatory cells and platelets, may play a significant role in PH.

Smooth Muscle Cells and Fibroblasts

A feature common to all forms of PH remodeling is the distal extension of smooth muscle into small peripheral, normally nonmuscular, pulmonary arteries within the respiratory acinus. In addition, a hallmark of severe PHis the formation of a layer of myofibroblasts and extracellular matrix between the endothelium and the internal elastic lamina, termed the neointima.There is good evidence to suggest that upregulation of matrix metalloproteinases (MMP2 and MMP9) occurs and that these molecules are involved in migration.[6]. In addition, evidence shows that PH may be associated with alterations of both rates of proliferation and apoptosis, which, in balance, result in thickened, obstructive pulmonary arteries.

Endothelial Cells

The initiating stimulus or injurythat results in abnormal endothelial proliferation is unknown,but may include hypoxia, shear stress, inflammation,or response to drugs or toxins on a background of geneticsusceptibility. Endothelial cells may respond to injury in various ways affecting theprocess of vascular remodeling. Injury can alter not only cell proliferation and apoptosis but also homeostatic functionsof the endothelium (including coagulation pathways, andproduction of growth factors and vasoactive agents). The cells comprising plexiform lesions are endothelial channels supported by a stroma containing matrix proteins and myofibroblasts. In addition, cells comprising plexiform lesions of idiopathic PH are monoclonal in origin [7].

Inflammatory Cells

Inflammatory mechanisms appear to play a significant role in some types of PH including monocrotaline-induced cases in rats and PH of various origins in humans including connective tissue diseases and human immunodeficiency virus infection [8]. A subset of PH patients have circulating autoantibodies including antinuclear antibodies, as well as elevated circulating levels of proinflammatory cytokines IL-1 and IL-6. Lung histology also revealed inflammatory infiltrates (macrophages and lymphocytes) in the range of plexiform lesions in severe PH as well as an increased expression of chemokines RANTES and fractalkine [9].

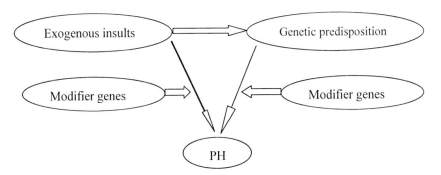

Figure 1. Paradigm for the "multiple-hit" hypothesis promoting pulmonary hypertension. Susceptible persons with genetic or acquired traits do not progressto pulmonary hypertension without suffering from additional insults that are synergistic in thepathogenesis of disease.

Platelets and Thrombosis

Thrombotic lesions and platelet dysfunction are potentially important processes in PH. Vascular abnormalities in PH may lead to release by platelets of various procoagulant, vasoactive, and mitogenic mediators. Indeed, in addition to its role in coagulation, the platelet stores and releases important contributors to pulmonary vasoconstriction and remodeling such as thromboxane A2, platelet activating factor, serotonin (5-hydroxytryptamine [5-HT]), platelet-derived growth factor (PDGF), TGF-β, and VEGF[10].

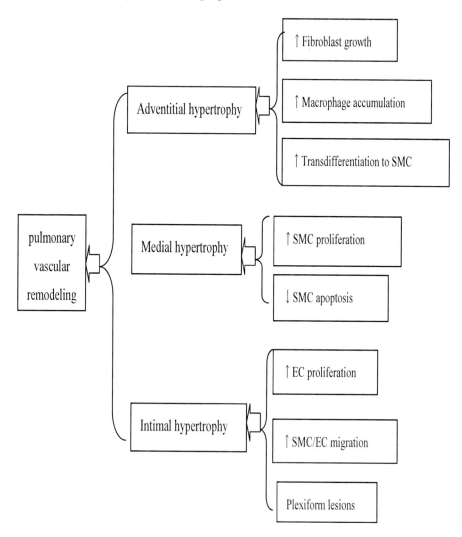

Figure 2. Cellular mechanisms of pulmonary vascular remodeling. SMC= pulmonary artery smooth muscle cell;EC= pulmonary artery endothelial cell; VSMC= pulmonary artery vascular smooth muscle cell.

Molecular Mechanisms

Genetic Association

Understanding of the mechanism of genetic predisposition to PH is of paramount importance for identification of the root pathogenesis. Mutations in the transforming growth factor-β receptor (TGF-β receptor) superfamily have been genetically linked to PH and likely play a causative role in the development of disease. A rare group of patients with hereditary hemorrhagic telangiectasia and idiopathic PH harbor specific mutations inALK1 or endoglin, genes encoding two such members of the TGF-β receptor superfamily [11,12]. However, a more prevalent cohort of patients carries mutations in another member, the bone morphogenetic protein receptor type 2 (BMPR2 gene which encodes for BMPR-II) [13,14]. Over 140 mutations in BMPR2 have been reported in patients with familial PH [15].

Acquired/Exogenous Factors

In addition to genetic predisposition, development of PH likely depends on a variety of physiologic, acquired, and/or exogenous stimuli. These include chronic hypoxia, hemoglobinopathies, autoimmune vascular disease, viral infections, congenital heart disease with systemic-to-pulmonary shunt, and "serotoninergic" anorexigen use, thrombocytosis, central nervous system stimulants, portal hypertension, persistent PH of the newborn, and female gender predilection.Acute hypoxia induces vasodilatation insystemic vessels, but induces vasoconstriction in pulmonary arteries. This acute and reversible effect is mediated in part by upregulation of vasoconstrictors, such as endothelin-1 and serotonin, and, in part, by hypoxia- and redox-sensitive potassium channel activity in pulmonary vascular smooth muscle cells. Coordinately, these events lead to membrane depolarization insmooth muscle cells, increase in cytosolic calcium, and vasoconstriction [16]. In contrast, chronic hypoxia induces vascular remodeling and less reversible changes, including migration and proliferation of vascular smooth muscle cells and deposition of extracellular matrix.PH is associated with hemoglobinopathies, especially thalessemias [17,18] and sickle cell anemia [19-21]. Hemolysis accompanying these disorders may lead to destruction of bioactive nitric oxide by free hemoglobin [22] or reactive oxygen species [23, 24]. Furthermore, reactive oxygen species may lead to increased levels of oxyhemoglobin, which further impairs the delivery of nitric oxide to the vessel wall.

Pulmonary arteriopathy complicates autoimmune diseases, especially in the setting of the CREST variant of limited systemic sclerosis and, to a lesser degree, in mixed connective tissue disease, systemic lupus erythematosis, and rheumatoid arthritis [25-28].

An association between the human immunodeficiency virus (HIV) infection and PHhas been noted in approximately 0.5% of all patients with HIV infection, a rate 6 to 12 times higher than the general population [29,30]. Mechanisms of disease have been proposed that directlystem from effects of HIV infection [31]. These include infection of smooth muscle cells with subsequent dysregulation of proliferation, imbalance of vascular mitogens in response to systemic HIV infection, and endothelial injury precipitated by HIV-infected T cells [32]. Recently, the direct actions of HIV-encoded proteins have been implicated in PHdevelopment. The HIV gp120 protein may induce pulmonary endothelial dysfunction and apoptosis [33]. Cell culture studies have also demonstrated a role for the HIV Tat protein in repression of BMPR-II transcription, potentially provoking a proliferative response in the vessel wall [34].

Increased flow through the pulmonary circulation has long been associated with development of PH. In contrast to the cases of unrestricted ventricular septal defect (VSD) and patent ductus arteriosus (PDA), only 10–20% of all persons with atrial septal defects (ASD) progress to PH [35]. This observation may reflect differences in the response of the pulmonary vasculature to pressure overload (as seen in shunts with VSD and PDA) ascompared to volume overload (as seen in shunts with ASD); A widely held hypothesis suggests that patients with ASD may harbor a specific, unidentified genetic predisposition to the development of PH that may work in concert with or independently of the increased volume load to the pulmonary circulation. At the molecular level, the physiologic flow patterns of laminar shear stress, turbulent flow, and cyclic strain are all recognized by endothelial cells, leading to transduction of intracellular signals and modulation of awide variety of phenotypic changes [36]. Recently, ex-vivo modeling of pulsatile flow with high levels of shear stress and chronic VEGF inhibition hasdemonstrated apoptosis of pulmonary artery endothelial cells followed by outgrowth and selection for proliferating apoptosis resistant cells [37]. Therefore, chronically elevated flow may allow for selection of cells with dysregulated endothelial cell growth and resulting clonal or polyclonal expansion to plexiformlesions.

Vascular Effectors

Downstream of the genetic and acquired triggers of PH, the histopathologic processes that predominate later stages of disease include vasoconstriction, cellular proliferation, and thrombosis. These processes are influenced by a complex and dysregulated balance of vascular effectors controlling vasodilatation and vasoconstriction, growth suppressors and growthfactors, and pro-versus antithrombotic mediators.(Table1).Gaseous vasoactive molecules regulate pulmonary vascular homeostasis, and alterations in their endogenous production have been linked to the progression of PH. Nitric oxide (NO) is a potent pulmonary arterial vasodilator as well as a direct inhibitor of platelet activation and vascular smooth muscle cell proliferation. The synthesis of NO is mediated by a family of NO synthase enzymes (NOS). The endothelial isoform (eNOS) is regulated by a multitude of vasoactive factors and physiologic stimuli, including hypoxia, inflammation, and oxidative stress. Reduced levels of eNOS have been demonstrated in the pulmonary vasculature of patients with PH, suggesting a mechanism of dysregulated vasoconstriction [38,39]. Correspondingly, a murine model that genetically lacks eNOS is more susceptible to developing PH in response to other endogenous stimuli, as compared with the wild type control [40,41]. Furthermore, the impact of NO has been reflected in its therapeutic role in PH, as shown by the clinical efficacy of inhaled NO [42] and the NO-dependent phosphodiesterase type-5 inhibitorsildenafil [43,44].

Carbon monoxide (CO) and hydrogen sulfide (H2S) are endogenously produced gaseous vasodilators, deficiencies of which may promote development of PH. Mice thatare null in heme-oxygenase-1 (HO-1), a primary enzyme that produces CO in the pulmonary vasculature, exhibit less tolerance for hypoxia with resulting right ventricular dysfunction [45]. In contrast, over expression of HO-1 in the lung prevents development of PH in murine models of chronic hypoxia [46] and in rat models of monocrotaline-induced PH [47]. H2S also functions as a vasodilator and inhibitor of vessel wall proliferation, which can protect against the development of PH in rat models [48,49].

The arachidonic acid metabolites prostacycl in and thromboxane A2 also play crucial roles in vasoconstriction, thrombosis, and, to a certain degree, vessel wall proliferation. Prostacyclin (prostaglandin I2) activates cyclic adenosinemonophosphate (cAMP)-dependent pathways and serves as a vasodilator, an antiproliferative agent for vascular smooth muscle, and an inhibitor of platelet activation and aggregation. In contrast, thromboxane A2 increases vasoconstriction and activates platelets [50]. Protein levels of prostacyclin synthaseare decreased in small and medium-sized pulmonary arteriesin patients with PH, particularly with the idiopathic form [51]. Biochemical analysis of urine in patients with PH hasshown decreased levels of a breakdown product of prostacyclin (6-keto-prostacyclin F2alpha), accompanied by increased levels of a metabolite of thromboxane A2 (thromboxane B2) [52].Recognition of this imbalance has led to the success of prostacyclin therapy and improvement of hemodynamics, clinical status, and survival inpatients with severe PH [53].

Endothelin-1 (ET-1) is expressed by pulmonary endothelial cells and has been identified as a significant vascular mediator in PH. It acts as both a potent pulmonary arterial vasoconstrictor and mitogen of pulmonary smooth muscle cells [54,55]. The vasoconstrictor response relies upon binding to the endothelin receptor A (ETA receptor) on vascular smooth muscle cells. This leads to an increase in intracellular calcium, along withactivation of protein kinase C, mitogen-activated protein kinase,and the early growth response genes c-fos and c-jun [56]. The resulting vasoconstriction, mitogenesis, and vascular remodeling arethought to lead to significant hemodynamic changes in the pulmonary vasculature and to PH. Plasma levels of endothelin-1 are increased in animal and human subjects suffering from PH due to a variety of etiologies [57,58]. Improvementin hemodynamics, clinical status, and survival of PH patients treated with chronic ET receptor antagonists highlights the significance of these effects [59].

Down regulation of vasoactive intestinal peptide (VIP) mayalso play a pathogenic role. VIP is a pulmonary vasodilator, aninhibitor of proliferation of vascular smooth muscle cells, and an inhibitor of platelet aggregation [60,61]. Decreased concentrationsof VIP have been reported in serum and lung tissue of patients with PH [63]. VIP-null mice suffer from moderate PH [64]. Furthermore, both pulmonary arterial pressure and pulmonary vascular resistance decrease after treatment with VIP [65]. Improvement of hemodynamics and clinical course has also been observed with inhaled VIP in a small number of PH patients [63].

Vascular endothelial growth factor (VEGF) is a well-studiedendothelial cell mitogen and angiogenic factor. In the pulmonary circulation, it binds endothelial cells via tyrosine kinase receptors.Production of VEGF and its receptors is upregulated in human pulmonary tissue in both acute and chronic hypoxia [66].Increased VEGF expression has also been observed in PH,accompanied by elevated levels of VEGFR-1 in the affected pulmonary endothelium and specifically elevated levels of VEGFR-2 in plexiform lesions [67]. As a result, a dysregulated responseto VEGF has been proposed to critically influence endothelialcell survival, proliferation, and apoptosis. Correspondingly, mice with homozygous deletions in the B isoform of VEGF (VEGF-B) demonstrate less vascular remodeling compared to wild type controls when exposed to hypoxia [68], indicating that VEGF-B can exacerbate vascular proliferative changes. Inrat models, a combination of chronic blockade of VEGFR-2 andhypoxia leads to pulmonary endothelial cell apoptosis and to the outgrowth of selected apoptosis-resistant, proliferating endothelial cells with severe PH [69].

It has been recently reported that peroxisome proliferator-activated receptor-rgamma (PPARγ) can ameliorate PH in insulin-resistant, apolipoprotein E-deficient mice [70]. This suggests not onlya link between insulin resistance/obesity and PH but also highlights a novel protective role for PPARγ in pulmonary vasculopathy.

Other potential contributing factors to PH progression include phosphordiesterase I [71], surviving [72], the calcium binding protein S100A4/Mts1 [73, 74], the transient receptor potential channels [75], and adrenomedullin [76-78]. Furthermore, other vascular growth factors such as platelet derived growth factor, basicfibroblast growth factor, insulin-like growth factor-1, and epidermal growth factor all may play down stream roles in later stages of PH. Insight into this topic is offered bythe fact that the above effectors are likely subject to upstream, over-arching regulatory pathways that affect the action of multiple vasoactive molecules [79]. Characterization of these regulatory mechanisms may eventually allow for identification of primary molecular triggers of disease and offer noveltherapeutic targets for drug development. Some examples of potential overarching and overlapping regulatory pathways may include those that function through rho-kinase, voltage activated potassium channels, angiopoietin-1, caveolae, 5-lipoxygenase (5-LO), and vascular elastase.

Multiple cell types in the vascular wall rely upon the rho-kinasesignaling pathway for homeostatic function and responseto injury [80]. These cell types include endothelial and vascular smooth muscle cells, inflammatory cells, and fibroblasts. Rho is a guanosine triphosphate (GTP) binding protein that activates its down stream target, rho-kinase, in response to activation of a variety of G-protein coupledreceptors. When activated, rho-kinase inhibits myosin phosphatase and conversely up regulates the ERM family of kinases. In vitro activation of these signaling cascades results in modulation of multiple cellular processes, including enhanced vasoconstriction, proliferation, impaired endothelial response to vasodilators,chronic pulmonary remodeling, and upregulation of vasoactive cytokines via the NF-κB transcription pathway.Rho-kinase activity has also been linked specifically to a number of known effectors of PH, including endothelin-1 [81, 82], serotonin [83, 84], and eNOS [85], among others. Recently, elevated rho-kinase activity has been demonstrated in animalmodels of PH [86, 87]. Furthermore, intravenous fasudil, aselective rho-kinase inhibitor, has induced pulmonary vasodilatation and regression of PH in various animal models [86-93]as well as in patients with severe PH who were otherwise refractory to conventional therapies [94, 95]. Interestingly, in amouse model of chronic hypoxia, PH improved after therapy with simvastatin, a 3-hydroxy-3-methylglutaryl CoA reductase inhibitor known also to inhibit rhokinaseactivity [96, 97]. Taken together, these data suggest that rho-kinase may control a master molecular "switch" in thepulmonary artery, initiating an activated state in disease from aquiescent state in health. As a result, rho-kinase represents anattractive and novel "upstream" therapeutic target for treatmentof PH.

Modulation of voltage-gated potassium channels (Kv) may also represent an overarching pathogenic mechanism of PH. Kv channels are inhibited in the smooth muscle cells of resistancevessels in the pulmonary arterial tree in response tohypoxia, and they regulate hypoxic pulmonary vasoconstriction [98]. Subsequent depolarization leads to theopening of voltage-gated calcium channels, an increase in intracellularcalcium, and the initiation of a number of intracellular signaling cascades promoting vasoconstriction and proliferationand inhibiting apoptosis. Expression array analysis has demonstrated a depletion of Kv1.5 channels in pulmonary tissuederived from PH patients [99]. Anumber of polymorphisms in the Kv1.5 channel gene (KCNA5) have been described, which may suggest a genetic predisposition to channel depletion. Appetite suppressants, such as dexfenfluramine and aminorex that are risk factors for development of PH, can also directly inhibit Kv1.5 and Kv2.1 [100].Inhibition of Kv currents in pulmonary smooth muscle cells maybe regulated by serotonin [101], thromboxane A2 [102], and,perhaps, nitric oxide [103]. Furthermore, BMP signaling can regulate Kv receptor expression [104,105]. Taken together, the Kv pathway may represent a common point of regulation in pathogenesis. Accordingly, augmentation of Kv activation would be predicted to induce vasodilatation and, perhaps, allow for regression of vessel remodeling. In vivo gene transfer of Kv channels in chronically hypoxic rats has led to improvement of PH and suggests its therapeutic potential [106].

Angiopoietin-1 is an angiogenic factor that has been linked tothe regulation of multiple vascular effectors of PH [107]. Angiopoietin-1 is produced by smooth muscle cellsand pericytes during vascular development; it binds the Tie2 receptor expressed on endothelium, which then activates smooth muscle proliferation and migration. After development, pulmonary expression is dramatically reduced; however, most nonfamilial forms of PH are characterized by up-regulation of

Tie2, and these levels correlate with severity of histologic disease. The level of angiopoietin-1 itself may also beupregulated in some cases [108,109]. In this context, angiopoietin-1 can stimulate pulmonary arterial endothelial cells to secrete mitogenic factors such as serotonin [110] and endothelin-1 [111]. It is conceivable that angiopoietin-1 mayserve as a crucial link between the serontoninergic and BMP pathways with resulting smooth muscle cell hyperplasia [112].In correlation, rodents expressing transgenic angiopoietin-1 inpulmonary tissue develop pulmonary vascular remodeling with diffuse smooth muscle cell hyperplasia in small pulmonary vessels. Furthermore, gene transfer of a Tie2 receptor antagonist ameliorates monocrotaline-induced PH in rats [110]. Paradoxically, angiopoietin-1 has also demonstrated aprotective role in some forms of PH, based on separate rodentstudies [113].

The actions of caveolae and its main coat protein caveolin-1(CAV-1) may also represent a possible upstream regulatory pathway of the development of PH. Caveolae are flask-shape dinvaginations found on the surface of the plasma membrane in avariety of vascular cell types, including pulmonary endothelium,vascular smooth muscle cells, and fibroblasts[114]. Caveolae are potential regulators of signaling functionthat spatially organize and concentrate signaling molecules.CAV-1 is depleted in plexiform lesions and muscularized pulmonary arterioles from patients with PH [115]. Furthermore, CAV-1-null mice develop a dilated cardiomyopathy and PH [116] with impaired NO and calcium signaling [117]. A number of possible pathogenic mechanisms can been visioned. Both eNOS [118] and endothelin-1 [119] are targeted to caveolae; disruption of these or other trafficking pathways could lead to increased inflammation and proliferation in thevessel wall [120]. BMPR-II may traffic through cholesterol-rich membrane rafts and caveolae, suggesting a possible regulatory role of caveolae for the BMP pathway and potential PH development [121]. Serotonin signaling may depend upon caveolae to downregulate Kv channels [122]. Moreover, CAV-1itself can function as a tumor suppressor gene, which, if depleted in the vasculature, may directly lead to increased proliferation [123].

A severe inflammatory state predominates end-staged PH and may play a significant role in pathogenesis. A number of soluble chemoattractants and pro-inflammatory cytokines from the pulmonary artery are upregulated in human and animal models of severe PH. These include interleukin-1β [124], transforming growth factor-β 1 [125], bradykinin [126], monocyte chemotactic protein-1 [127], fractalkine [128], RANTES [129], and leukotrienes [130], among others. 5-lipoxygenase (5-LO) regulates the synthesis of leukotrienes, which in turn can promote cytokine release. 5-LO may represent a possibleupstream factor involved in inciting this pro-inflammatory state [131]. 5-LO promotes endothelial cell proliferation in cellculture, and elevated levels of 5-LO have been detected inmacrophages and pulmonary endothelium derived from patients suffering from idiopathic PH [132]. In both a monocrotaline treated rat model [133] and a genetically susceptible BMPR2 +/−heterozygote mouse model of PH, overexpression of 5-LO via adenoviral delivery has worsened PH and vascular remodeling. Furthermore, 5-LO inhibitors have attenuated PH in both of these models. It is tempting to speculate that 5-LO may possess an upstream regulatory role in PH progression.

Table 2. Dysregulation of vascular effectors in pulmonary hypertension

Vascular effector	Change in activity in PH	Effect on vasoconstriction	Effect on cell proliferation	Effect on thrombosis
Serotonin	Increased	Increased	Increased	Increased
Nitric oxide	Decreased (increased in plexiform lesions)	Increased	(?) Increased in plexiform lesions	Increased
Thromboxane A2	Increased	Increased	Increased	Increased
Prostacyclin	Decreased	Increased	Increased	Increased
Endothelin-1	Increased	Increased	Increased	(N/A)
Vasoactive intestinal peptide (VIP)	Decreased	Increased	Increased	Increased
Vascular endothelial growth factor (VEGF)	Increased	(N/A)	Increased	(N/A)
Rho-kinase	Increased	Increased	Increased	Increased
Kv channel	Decreased	Increased	Increased	(N/A)
Angiopoietin-1	Increased	(N/A)	Increased	(N/A)
Caveolae	Decreased	(?)	(?)	(?)
5-Lipoxygenase (5-LO)	Increased	Increased	Increased	Increased
Vascular elastas	Increased	Increased	Increased	Increased

An imbalance of mediators of pulmonary vascular response has been observed in PH. Less significant effects are denoted by (N/A); unclear effects are indicated by (?).

Vascular-specific serine elastase activity has been implicated in the pathogenesis of PH via regulation of the remodeling response in the extracellular matrix [134]. In pulmonary arterioles, serine elastases are secreted into the extracellular space to activate matrix metalloproteinases (MMP) and to inhibit tissue inhibitors of MMP (TIMP). Both MMP and elastases degrade most components of the extracellular matrix leading to an upregulation of fibronect in and subsequent enhancement of cellular migration. Matrix degradation also leads to increased integrin signaling with resulting expression of the glycoprotein tenascin C. Tenascin C actscooperatively with other growth factors (i.e., epidermal growth factor) to enhance smooth muscle proliferation. Increased degradation of elastin [135] has been observed in pulmonary arteries from patients suffering from congenital heart disease and resultant pulmonary hypertension. In addition, rat models of PH have demonstrated increased productionand activity of vascular elastases [136] and tenascin C [137].Tenascin C also is induced in pulmonary tissue of patientsharboring BMPR2 mutations and suffering from familial PH [138]. This upregulation of elastase function may be induced bya number of vascular effectors implicated in PH, including NO [139], serotonin [140], and theoretically, the BMP pathway.Elastase inhibitors can induce apoptosis of smooth muscle cellsin cell culture and can improve PH in animal models [141-143].

Diagnosis

Screening

Patients with complaints of dyspnea on exertion and chest pain, with or without dizziness, syncope, and signs of right heart failure of unknown cause, should be screened for PH. Chest X-rays and electrocardiography (ECG) can be employed in PH screening programs.

ECG

In patients with PH, ECG can show increased P wave amplitude ($\geq$ 2.5 mm in the DII derivation), signs of right ventricular hypertrophy, right bundle branch block, right QRS axis deviation, and repolarization changes (right ventricular strain). Although a deviation greater than 100° has been shown to correlate well with hemodynamic measurements, its specificity for the diagnosis of PH has been shown to be low. Up to 13% of the patients with a diagnosis of PH confirmed by right heart catheterization (RHC) can initially present with normal ECG results. [144]

Chest X-ray

A chest X-ray reveals hilar enlargement that reflects pulmonary artery dilation and cardiomegaly. Chest X-rays also play an important role in the diagnosis of other diseases, such as those that impair the lung parenchyma and can cause dyspnea.

Chest CT

Computed angiotomography of the chest plays a significant role in the diagnostic evaluation of PH. The diameter of the PA trunk is significantly larger in patients with PH than in normal individuals and correlates well with PA pressure measurements. [145]Studies have shown that the diameter of the PA ranges from 32.6 mm to 33.2 mm in normal individuals. One811group of authors found that a PA diameter > 33.2 mm has a 95% specificity for the diagnosis of PH. [146]

Echocardiography

Echocardiography is the principal screening tool for PH. However, echocardiography is a test that has significant limitations, such as the fact that it is highly examiner-dependent and that a significant proportion of patients present with a poor acoustic window. Another limitation of echocardiography is that the estimation of PA systolic pressure (PASP) depends on the tricuspid regurgitant jet and right atrial pressure (RAP). In up to 10% of cases, it is impossible to measure the tricuspid regurgitant jet velocity and, consequently, to estimate PASP. Although some studies have shown a significant correlation between echocardiography findings and right heart catheterization values, one group of authors recently reported that the RAP and PASP values estimated by echocardiography differ significantly from those measured by right heart catheterization [147].In that study, 65 patients referred for PH diagnosis or follow-up treatment underwent echocardiography and right heart catheterization one hour apart, meaning that the basal conditions of patients varied minimally. It was also shown that cardiac output as measured by echocardiography is not useful and that echocardiography typically overestimates pressures. Therefore, PASP values as estimated by echocardiography should be used to screen for PH, rather than to diagnose it. In addition to PASP estimates, dilation and right ventricular dysfunction should be considered to constitute indirect signs of PH. Despite its limitations, echocardiography continues to be the principal screening tool for PH because it is a noninvasive and readily available test, as well as being useful in identifying left heart malformations and diseases.

Because right ventricular function plays a significant role in the prognosis of patients with PH, it is necessary to measure right ventricular function appropriately. The characteristics of the right ventricle (RV) are quite different from those of the left ventricle (LV). Unlike the LV, which has thick, cone-shaped walls, the RV has thin, semilunar or crescent-shaped walls, and the myocardial mass of the RV is significantly lower and more trabecular than is that of the LV. The contraction pattern is also different; in the RV, longitudinal contraction of the myocardial fibers predominates, whereas, in the LV, spiral movement predominates. Therefore, it does not seem sufficient or appropriate to evaluate right ventricular function with the same tools used to evaluate left ventricular function.

New techniques for a better estimation of right ventricular function have been studied. The determination of tricuspid annular plane systolic excursion (TAPSE) has been shown to be a useful tool. This technique calculates the degree to which the pulmonary valve ring is shifted, in relation to the right ventricular apex during systole. A study comparing TAPSE and RHC measurements for the evaluation of right ventricular function showed that the measurements correlated well. The authors found that a TAPSE < 1.8 cm showed good accuracy in detecting right ventricular dysfunction and designated it a prognostic marker, because survival rates were lower in patients with a TAPSE < 1.8 cm than in those with a TAPSE ≥ 1.8 cm.[148]

Magnetic Resonance Imaging

Advances in the techniques for acquiring and processing magnetic resonance imaging of the797heart have allowed three-dimensional evaluation of the RV and detailed tomographic visualization of its morphology. Cardiac magnetic resonance imaging (CMRI) creates a clear distinction between the myocardium and intracavitary blood, presenting well-defined myocardial and endocardial borders. [149] Because the RV presents the aforementioned particularities and CMRI allows a more detailed visualization of the RV, CMRI is currently considered the gold standard for a noninvasive evaluation of the RV. [150, 151]Studies in which CMRI was used to evaluate patients with PH showed that, when compared with control group patients, PH patients presented with a significant increase in end-systolic and end-diastolic volumes, as well as in right ventricular muscle mass, together with a significant reduction in right ventricular ejection fraction. Other studies have shown ventricular septal bowing, together with a reduction in the LV volume in early diastole, revealing impaired left ventricular function associated with right ventricular dysfunction. [152] One group of authors demonstrated that the position of the septum, as determined by calculating its shift toward the LV, was accurate in predicting right ventricular systolic pressure. [153] Even without the use of contrast enhancement, CMRI allows excellent visualization of the PA, and it is possible to assess PA compliance and flow by means of the phase-contrast technique. In patients with PH, PA compliance values are significantly lower. [154] One study showed that measurements of pulsatility (which is related to compliance) can also correlate with the response to the NO test. [155] The measurement of PA velocity and the time it takes to reach the maximum velocity (acceleration time) are reduced in patients with PH, and these measurements are related to systolic volume as measured by RHC. [156] In addition, CMRI plays a role in the follow-up of patients with PH. Two studies used CMRI before treatment initiation and 6-12 months after treatment initiation. In one of the studies, the patients received epoprostenol, and in the other, they received bosentan. [157,158] In both studies, improvement in the six-minute walk test was significantly related to improvement in right ventricular function parameters, as determined by CMRI. In another study, CMRI was used before and after pulmonary thromboendarterectomy. [159] The study showed a significant reduction in myocardial mass, right ventricular end-systolic volume, and right ventricular end-diastolic volume, as well as increased left ventricular volumes, reflecting the reversion of ventricular remodeling and septal deviation, hemodynamic improvement having been achieved with the surgical procedure.

Although CMRI is not widely available and its cost is still high, the role of CMRI in the diagnosis and follow-up of patients with PH is promising, because the test allows a better evaluation of right ventricular function, PA flow, and PA behavior.

If a patient suspected of having PH has been screened and signs consistent with increased pressure levels in the pulmonary circulation have been detected in the initial tests, the needto perform RHC to confirm the diagnosis of PH should be evaluated, because a definitive diagnosis of PH can only be established by invasive pressure measurements.

The acute test with a vasodilator should be performed during the initial hemodynamic evaluation in patients with PH. The test can be performed with NO, prostacyclin, or adenosine. The result is considered positive when there is a reduction in the MPAP of $\geq$ 10 mmHgand when values $\leq$ 40 mmHg are observed. A positive acute test result predicts the clinical and hemodynamic response to calcium channel blockers. [160, 161]

Treatments

The treatment of Pulmonary hypertension—once a lethal condition—has evolved considerably over the past few years as the number of therapeutic options available to treat this disease has increased, including calcium-channel blockers, prostacyclin and its analogs, phosphodiesterase type 5 inhibitors, endothelin-receptor antagonists and combination therapy, The novel emerging therapies, such as imatinib, fasudil, simvastatin, ghrelin and vasoactive intestinal peptide, hold therapeutic potential for disease modification as well as treatment of symptoms.

General Measures and Supportive Therapy

All patients diagnosed with PH should receive some general instructions. The patients should be instructed not to do heavy physical exercise and to limit physical activity when experiencing mild dyspnea. They should receive influenza vaccination and pneumococcal vaccination because infection is a major cause of morbidity and mortality in these patients. Female patients of childbearing age should be instructed to use contraceptive methods, because pregnancy significantly increases mortality in patients with PH. Although there is no consensus regarding theideal type of contraception for patients with PH, it should be borne in mind that concomitant use of bosentan and oral contraceptives can reduce the effect of the latter. Patients in functional class III or IV, as well as those with hypoxemia (PaO2 < 60 mmHg), should use supplemental oxygen if flying or visiting areas at altitudes above 1,500-2,000 m. [162]

Supplemental oxygen therapy is indicated for patients with hypoxemia (PaO2 < 60 mmHg) and can be considered for patients who present symptomatic benefit from the correction of hypoxemia during physical exertion. The use of diuretics is indicated for all patients who present with signs of hypervolemia. [162]

The use of anticoagulants in patients with PH is controversial, because there have been no randomized controlled studies evaluating the effects of anticoagulation in these patients. The rationale for the indication of anticoagulation for these patients originates from the histopathological findings of microvascular thrombosis, activation of the coagulation system, and platelet dysfunction in patients with IPH, which have led to the assumption that these patients present with a prothrombotic state. In a meta-analysis of the theme, conducted in 2006, the authors concluded that anticoagulation should be indicated, given that 5 of the 7 studies analyzed demonstrated that anticoagulation was beneficial. In the absence of any contraindications, the use of oral anticoagulants is indicated for patients with PH, with the objective of maintaining an international normalized ratio of 1.5-2.5. Attention should be given to patients with liver disease and scleroderma, because these patients might be at a higher risk for bleeding; likewise, attention should be given to the interaction between anticoagulants and the PH-specific treatment. Some studies, for instance, have suggested that concomitant use of anticoagulants and sitaxsentan can increase the risk of bleeding.[163]

Calcium-Channel Blockers

Patients who might respond to long-term therapywith calcium-channel blockers (CCBs) are identifiedby their initial response to a vasodilator challenge. [160, 161]Vasodilator testing is typically performed with potent, short-acting, titratablevasodilators such as nitric oxide, [161] prostacyclin and adenosine. If the response is positive the patient could benefit from CCB therapy. The CCBs predominantly used are nifedipineand diltiazem. Amlodipine is also effectiveand is increasingly used. [162, 163] Notably, only approximately10–15% of patients with IPH will meet the criteria for a positive response, and only half of those will receive sustained clinical and hemodynamic benefits. [164]

Anticoagulation

In the absence of any contraindication, anticoagulationwith warfarin is generally recommendedon the basis of findings from retrospective,single-center studies that indicated an improvedsurvival in those with IPH. [165] Aspirin andclopidogrel in combination with epoprostenolcould improve platelet function parameters inpatients with PH. [166]

Prostacyclin Therapy

In patients with a negative vasodilator challengeresult, severe PH and evidence of right ventriculardysfunction, therapy with chronic intra -venous epopro stenol should be considered. Presently, epopro stenol seems to be the most potenttreatment available for this group of patients, although no findings from direct comparison trials with other agents are available. Although epoprostenol produces an acute hemodynamic effect insome patients,most patients experience longterm benefit despite the absence of any acute hemodynamicchange. This benefit could be secondary toan effect on pulmonary vascular remodeling. [167] Aninitial 3-month prospective, open, randomized trialdemonstrated that epoprostenol improved hemodynamic characteristics, exercise tolerance, qualityof life, and survival in patients in NYHA functionalclasses III and IV compared with a similar groupof patients who received conventional therapy (i.e.diuretics, cardiac glycosides, oral vasodilators andanticoagulants). [168] Of note, the dose of prostacyclin has to be increased on a regular basis, possiblybecause of tachyphylaxis, and administration canproduce pulmonary edema in patients with venoocclusive disease. Furthermore, acute withdrawal ofthe medication can result in rebound PH, which can be fatal. Other adverse effects include jaw pain, cutaneous and gastrointestinal symptoms, and myalgias and foot or leg pain.Studies of patients with PH treated with epoprostenol have shown a survival of about 65% after 3 years. [169, 170] Although long-term follow-updata exist on the use of intravenous epoprostenol, in the present era this drug is no longer the first choice agent because of the availability of newer oral agents, which are usually tried first. Epoprostenol tends to be reserved as therapy for patients who present with severe hemodynamic compromise.

Prostacyclin Analogs

The effects of continuous subcutaneous administration of the synthetic prostacyclin analog treprostinilin patients with PH were studied in a large randomized controlled trial, and improvementsin exercise capacity, hemodynamics and clinicalevent rate were demonstrated. [171] In this study of 470 patients, the treprostinil-treated group demonstrated no deterioration in 6 min walk test distance,whereas the placebo-treated group did show adecrease from baseline to week 12 ($P = 0.06$).Although there was no significant difference inmean PAP between the two treatment groups,there was a significant decrease in the PVR indexwith treprostinil therapy ($P = 0.0002$). The adverseeffects reported included the presence of pain at theinjection site, and 8% of patients discontinued the medication. An additional controlled pilot studywas performed with treprostinil in 26 patients with PH and showed trends in the improvement of6 min walk test and in the reduction of PVR. [172] An initial pilot studyand a subsequent small randomized controlledtrial of intravenous treprostinil concluded thatlong-term intra venous infusion of this agent wassafe and effective for the treatment of patients with PH.[173] As with subcutaneous treprostinil, intravenous streprostinil has been approved for use inthe US but is not widely available in Europe.A study of aerosolized iloprost in 35 patientswith PH demonstrated that a 14–17 mg dose of this agent was more potent than 40 ppm of inhaled nitric oxide as a pulmonary vasodilator. [174]Subsequently, inhaled iloprost was evaluated in a randomized controlled trial that enrolled patientswith PH and compared this agent with placebo.The study showed that iloprost increased exercise capacity and improved symptoms, PVR, and time to clinical events in patients with IPH. Hoeper *et al.* showed that a single inhalation of iloprostresulted in a 10–20% reduction in mean PAP,lasting for 45–60 min. [174] A long-term uncontrolled study of 25 patients with PH treated with inhaled iloprost for at least 1 year showed an increasein 6 min walk test distance of 85 m, a reduction in mean PAP of 7 mmHg and an increase in cardiacindex of 0.6 l/min/m2.[175]One potential advantage of this medication compared with intravenousepoprostenol is that iloprost might cause lessventilation– perfusion mismatch; however, thelong-term efficacy of inhaled iloprost has yet tobe established. Beraprost is an oral prostacyclin analog that showed some benefit in an initial pilot study,[176]and two randomized controlled trials. [177]

Nitric Oxide

NO stimulates guanylate cyclase to generate cyclic GMP, which mediates vasodilation and inhibits smooth muscle cell proliferation. Because it combines the advantages of potent pulmonary vasodilation, virtual absence of systemic effects, by virtue of its immediate inactivation by hemoglobin, and ability to improve oxygenation like other inhaled agents, some have considered inhaled NO the "drug of choice" for intraoperative pulmonary hypertension. [178] It offers a safety margin, and with a commercially available delivery device (INO Therapeutics, Clinton, New Jersey) is easy to administer and titrate, either via mechanical ventilator or face mask. Numerous case reports and small series and a few randomized trials have been reported on its application for acute right heart syndrome, both in the postoperative setting and otherwise. While INO has been shown to be of benefit in reducing the PVR of acute pulmonary hypertension, independent of cause [179], its effects in patients with chronic PHT are less predictable. Although some patients with chronic PHT do show an acute vasodilator response to INO, others do not [180, 181]. This most likely relates to the relative degree of medial hypertrophy versus intimal hyperplasia and luminal thrombosis that occurs in the small pulmonary arteries in chronic lung vascular disease. Because of its potency and rapid onset of action, INO has been suggested as a screening tool for defining which patients with pulmonary hypertension may benefit from long term [180, 181]. In these studies which used invasive haemodynamic monitoring, there was a strong correlation be tween response to INO and subsequent response to oral therapy. Because only 30–40% of the subjects respond to INO [180-182], this finding represents a significant step forward in directed therapy. An attempt to assess the response to INO using a 6-min walk as a non-invasive marker of reversibility of pulmonary hypertension was not successful in a small clinical trial [183]. In that study of 6 patients, there was no significant difference in distance walked or symptoms experienced during INO compared to placebo. Occasional patients with PHT who do have a vasodilator response have been 'bridged' to transplantation with INO for as long as 68 days. Inhaled NO may also have a role in 'bridging' patients with a degree of fixed pulmonary hypertension during periods of acute pulmonary decompensation.

Table 3. Established therapeutic options for pulmonary hypertension

Drug	Administration	Typical dose	Adverse effects
Nifedipine	Oral	120–240 mg qd	Hypotension, peripheral edema
Diltiazem	Oral	240–720 mg qd	Hypotension, peripheral edema
Amlodipine	Oral	10–40 mg qd	Hypotension, peripheral edema
Epoprosteno	Continuous IV infusion	10–15 ng/kg/min	Jaw pain, cutaneous or gastrointestinal symptoms and myalgias
Trepostinil	SC or IV infusion	5–15 ng/kg/min	Erythemas, site pain at SC infusion site
Iloprost	Inhaled	30–150 μg qd	Jaw pain, myalgias
Beraprost	Oral	60–200 μg qd	Headache, flushing
Bosentan	Oral	250 mg qd	Hepatotoxicity, peripheral edema
Sitaxentan	Oral	300 mg qd	Flushing, hepatotoxicity, warfarin interaction
Ambrisentan	Oral	2.5–10.0 mg qd	Flushing
Sildenafil	Oral	20 mg tid	Hypotension, shortness of breath, interaction with nitrates
Tadalafil	Oral	20–50 mg qd	Headache, dyspepsia
warfarin	Oral	2–10 mg qd	Bleeding
Supportive therapy			
Oxygen	Intermittent or continuous inhalation	NA	NA
Furosemide	Oral	20–100 mg qd	Hypotension
Digoxin	Oral	0.125–0.50 mg qd	Arrhythmias, vomiting
Inotropes (dopamine, dobutamine, milrinone)	IV	See individual agents	Tachycardia
ACE inhibitors and angiotensin-receptor blockers	Oral	See individual agents	Hypotension

IV, intravenous; NA, not available; ND, no data; PDEI, phosphodiesterase type 5 inhibitor; PDGF, platelet-derived growth factor; PH, pulmonary hypertension; qd, once daily.

Phosphodiesterase Type 5 inhibitors

Sildenafil is an oral selective inhibitor of cyclic- GMP-specific phosphordiesterase type 5, which exerts its effects by increasing intracellular cyclic GMP levels. This increase induces relaxation of and has antiproliferative effects on vascular smooth muscle cells. [184] A number of small, largely uncontrolled studies have reported favorable effects of sildenafil in patients with PH. [185-189] The findings of a pivotal randomized controlled trial of 278 patients with PH in NYHA classes II and III showed improved 6 min walk test distances and reduced mean PAP after 12 weeks with sildenafil. [190] A study of tadalafil (a newer phospho diesterase type 5 inhibitor that acts longer than sildenafil) also showed a favorable patient outcome, indicating that tadalafil could also be useful in the treatment of PH. [191]

Endothelin -Receptorantagonists

Endothelin-1 levels are significantly elevated inpatients with PH. A powerful rationale, therefore, exists for the use of endothelin-receptor antagonists.[192] Endothelin-1 induces vasoconstriction andmyocyte hypertrophy, and concentration correlates with PH severity and prognosis. Furthermore, endothelin-1 receptors are highly expressed in the plexiform lesions in PH. [193] Endothelin receptors consist of two subtypes. The endothelin- A (ETA) receptor is responsible for smooth muscle vasoconstriction and proliferation. ETA receptor stimulation causes increased inotropic activity, as oconstriction and smooth-muscle-cell proliferation. Stimulation of endothelin-B (ETB) receptors on endothelial cells, on the other hand, has antagonistic actions and results in nitric oxidea nd prostacyclin release as well as increased endothelin clearance, but stimulation of ETB receptorsin smooth muscle cells also provokes proliferation and vasoconstriction. [194-196] For this reason, it is unclear whether selective ETA receptor blockade is advantageous compared with dual blockade of both the ETA and ETB receptors. The orally administered, dual endothelin-receptor antagonist bosentan has been evaluated in randomized controlled trials that have shown improvement in exercise capacity, NYHA class, hemodyamics, echocardiographic and Doppler variables, and time toclinical worsening in patients with PH. [197,198] Onthe basis of these results, in the US bosentan has been approved for the treatment of NYHA class III and IV patients with PH (only class III patientsare approved to receive treatment in Europe). The most significant adverse effect of bosentanis liver function abnormality, which occurs inapproximately 12% of patients. [195] Sitaxentan is an endothelin-receptor antagonist that is significantly more selective for the ETA than the ETB receptor. This agent has been assessed in a randomized controlled trial of 178 patients with PH (NYHA class II, III or IV), and improved patients'exercise capacity, hemodynamics and clinicalevent rates. [199] Another controlled trial randomly allocated 247 patients with PH to placebo (n = 62), 50 mg sitaxentan (n = 62) or 100 mgsitaxentan daily (n = 61). After 18 weeks, patients treated with 100 mg sitaxentan had improved 6 min walk test distance (P = 0.03) and NYHA class (P = 0.04) compared with placebo-treatedpatients. [200] Sitaxentan has been approved for usein Europe and Australia and is under consideration for approval in the US. Ambrisentan (currently inphase III trials) is another selective ETA receptor antagonist, with favorable pharmacokinetics and good safety profile. [201] Thus far ambrisentan has been reported only in a blinded, dose-comparison pilot study in 64 patients with PH. In a doseranging study after 12 weeks, ambrisentan significantly improved 6 min walk test distance, NYHA class and mean PAP. Mild adverse events, including elevated liver enzyme levels, were present in only3% of patients.53 Importantly, unlike sitaxentan, ambrisentan has no drug interactions, especiallywith warfarin-type anticoagulants. [199] (Table 3).

Combination Therapy

As different factors contribute to the development and progression of PH, the disease should be approached from different therapeutic angles. Data supporting this concept are accumulating and consideration should be given to a combination therapy approach started early. The efficacy and safety of the combination of bosentan and epoprostenol were investigated in a study of 33 patients with severe PH enrolled in a placebo-controlled, prospective study.93 Although improved hemodynamics, exercise capacity and NYHA class were observed in both groups, the data showed a trend for a greater improvement in all hemodynamic parameters in the combination-treatment group than in the placebo-treatment group. [202] The data concerning inhaled iloprost and bosentan is less clear; uncontrolled studies have demonstrated variable results. [203,204] Two randomized controlled trials have also provided mixed results, with one study failing to show an improvement 94 and the other study indicating that the combination is safe and possibly effective. [205] The difficulties of assessing the results of these studies have been highlighted in an editorial by Gomberg-Maitland, [206] which accompanied the study from Hoeper *et al*.94 This editorial suggested that the difficulty could relate in part to the severity of illness of some of the patients entering these studies. Wilkens and colleagues found that the addition of sildenafil to inhaled iloprost was beneficial in reducing mean PAP and enhanced the latter agent's effect. [207] There could also be benefit from combining subcutaneous treprostinil with sildenafil, [208] implying that oral sildenafil could also enhance the effect of intravenous epoprostenol. Another logical combination would be bosentan and sildenafil; animal studies have shown that this combination has an incremental effect in decreasing PAP, reducing plasma catecholamine levels, maintaining body weight and reducing mortality risk. [209, 210]Similarly, the combination of bosentan and tadalafil could prove effective. [211] Further studies are planned or ongoing to evaluate the therapeutic potential of various combination therapies.

Management of PH associated with Congenital Systemic-to-pulmonary Shunts and Eisenmenger's Syndrome

A large proportion of patients with congenital heart disease (CHD), in particular those with relevant systemic-to-pulmonary shunts, will develop PH if left untreated. Eisenmenger's syndrome, the most advanced form of PH associated with CHD, is defined as CHD with an initial large systemic-to-pulmonary shunt that induces severe pulmonary vascular disease and PH, with resultant reversal of the shunt and central cyanosis. [212]

The treatment strategy for patients with PH associated with congenital systemic-to-pulmonary shunts and, in particular, those with Eisenmenger's syndrome is based mainly on clinical experience rather than being evidence based. Lung transplantation with repair of the cardiac defect or combined heart-lung transplantation is option for patients with Eisenmenger's syndrome who have indicators of a poor prognosis (syncope, refractory right-sided heart failure, NYHA functional class III or IV or severe hypoxaemia). [213] Because of the somewhat limited success of transplantation and the reasonably good survival of patients treated medically, careful selection of patients for transplantation is imperative.

Novel Speculative Therapies

A summary of all novel, emerging therapiesexamined here can be found in Table 4.

Rho-kinase Inhibitor: Fasudil

Rhokinase-mediated calcium sensitization is centralin mediating the sustained vasoconstriction and increased vasoreactivity in the rat hypoxic model of PH, [214] which when treated with the Rho-kinaseinhibitor fasudil exhibits reduced PAP. [215] The first clinical study with intravenous fasudil enrolled nine patients with severe PH and found that fasudil treatment caused a slight decrease in the mean PAP along with an increase in the cardiac index, though neither response was significant. Fasudildid, however, cause a significant decrease in PVR. [216]In theory, the beneficial effect of phosphodiesterasetype 5 inhibitors, such as sildenafil, could in part be mediated by Rho-kinase inhibition. [217]

PDGF Receptor Antagonist: Imatinib

PDGF has been implicated in endothelial cell dysfunction and proliferation and migration of vascular smooth muscle cells, which in turn might be involved in the vascular remodeling observed in PH. [218] Furthermore, PDGF is implicated in chronic myeloproliferative disorders (including myelofibrosis) that are associated with a high incidence of PH, [219] which indicates that bone marrow fibrosis could be associated in part with the development of PH. [220] Imatinib, a PDGF receptor antagonist approved for the treatment of chronicmyeloid leukemia, has been used in patients with PH. An animal study showed reversal of pulmonary vascular remodeling and improvement of PH with imatinib. [221] In an initial case report ofits use in a patient already receiving combination therapy, the patient showed improved 6-min walk test distance, hemodynamics and NYHA class after 3 months of imatinib treatment. Follow up after 6 months of treatment revealed sustained clinical efficacy. [222] Further case reports have followed since, implying imatinib's efficacy in cases of severe PH. [223, 224] Toxic effects on the heart,however, could be an adverse effect of long-termuse, which might limit its utility. [225]

Simvastatin

A study of simvastatin demonstrated improvementin the bone morphogenetic protein receptortype-2 signaling pathway in pulmonary artery smooth muscle and lung microvascular endothelial cells. [226]Although further studies are needed, this finding indicates that simvastatin could enhance endothelial function. Simvastatin might also be effective in inducing apoptosis in hyper proliferative pulmonary vascular lesions. [227] A small study of 16 patients reported improvements in 6 min walk tests in patients receiving 20–80 mg of simvastatindaily. [228]

Ghrelin

Other emerging therapeutic possibilities include ghrelin, an endogenous vasodilatory peptide that also stimulates the release of growth hormone, and has been demonstrated to attenuate the development of PH in a monocrotaline treated animal model of PH. [229]

Bradykinin

Bradykinin is apotent modulator of endothelial-cell function and a study of a stable bradykinin receptor agonist has demonstrated bradykinin's capacity to reduce severe PH and right ventricular hypertrophy. [230].This study also showed bradykinin could induce apoptosis of hyperproliferative cells through endothelial nitric oxide activation and induction of prostacyclin production.PH is associated with increased lung expression of the 5-hydroxy tryptamine transporter, which promotes smooth-muscle-cell proliferation. [231] and could potentially be involved in the development of PH.

Fluoxetine

Subtypes of the 5-hydroxy tryptamine receptor could also be involved in the pathogenesisof PH and are being targeted in PH treatment. [232]The selective 5-hydroxy tryptamine transporter inhibitor fluoxetine has been shown to prevent or reverse PH in a monocrotaline animal modelof PH, [233] and could form the basis of a potential future therapeutic strategy in humans.Vasoactive intestinal peptide (a neuro peptide with a potent bronchodilator, systemic andpulmonary vasodilator properties[234]) has been shown to be decreased in the serum and lung tissue of patients with PH. [235] When administered in aerosol form, it improved hemodynamic parameters without adverse effects in a small pilot study of eight patients.[235] Longer-term studies willbe necessary to assess the therapeutic potential of this agent. In monocrotaline-induced PH, disease progression isassociated with increased lung expression of the serotonin transporter, which promotes the proliferation of pulmonary artery smooth muscle cells. The selective serotonin transporter inhibitor fluoxetine prevented or reversed PH in this model [236]. Considering the good safety profile and wide use of fluoxetine in humans as an antidepressant, a PH RCT is justified, However, arecent trial suggested that maternal fluoxetine (taken in the third trimester) increases the risk of primary PH of the newborn [237].

Potassium Channel Augmentation

The voltage-gated potassium channel might also have a role in the pathogenesis of pulmonary hypertension, interacting with endothelin-1 aswell as 5-hydroxy tryptamine. Studies of voltagegated potassium-channel over expression achieved by nebulized adenoviral Kv1.5 gene therapy or oral dichloroacetate can regress experimental PH and could have therapeutic potential. A common feature in experimental [238,239] and human PH [240] is the decreased expression of voltage-gated potassium channels, particularly Kv1.5. The loss of potassium channels causes membrane depolarization and increases cytosolic calcium, thereby promoting vasoconstriction and cell proliferation. In addition, the loss of these channels increases cytosolic potassium concentrations, which inhibits caspases and reduces apoptosis [241]. Potassium channel overexpression (whether achieved by nebulized adenoviral Kv1.5 gene therapy [238] or oral dichloroacetate) can regress experimental PH.

Apoptosis Signal-Regulating Kinase 1

Apoptosis signal-regulating kinase 1 (ASK1) is a member of mitogen-activated protein kinase kinase kinase (MAPKKK) family and is activated in response to TNF-a, Fas, and H2O2[242]. Activation of ASK1 in turn leads to activation of MAPKs such as JNK and p38 and results inapoptosis [243]. ASK1 plays a critical role in vascular remodeling, directly participating in VSMC (vascular smooth muscle cell) proliferation and migration and neointimal thickening in injured artery. ASK1 may provide the basis for the development of new therapeutic strategies forvascular diseases [244].

Peroxisome Proliferator-Activated Receptor Gamma

The peroxisome proliferator-activated receptor gamma (PPARgamma) is a member of the nuclear hormonereceptor superfamily of ligand-activated transcription factors.Transcriptional activation of the PPARgamma receptor requires heterodimerization with the retinoid Xreceptor (RXR). Activation of the receptor is promoted bystructurally diverse ligands, including thiazolidinediones (TZDs) and long-chain fatty acids and their metabolites.Among these ligands, the synthetic TZD class, includingrosiglitazone and pioglitazone, has been used for clinicalbenefit in patients with type 2 diabetes where these medicationsenhance insulin sensitivity and reduce metabolicderangements [245].PPARgamma is expressed in the lung and pulmonary vasculature, and its expression is reduced in the vascularlesions of patients with PH. Furthermore, ligands for PPARgamma reduced vascular remodeling in rat and mouse models of PH. Ligands for PPARgamma have been shown to attenuate proliferation of vascular smooth muscle cells and to induce apoptosis in several cell lines invitro [246,247]. PPARgamma ligands reduce monocrotaline induced PH and pulmonary vascular wall thickening inrats by inhibiting monocrotaline-induced cell proliferation and inducing apoptosis in the pulmonary arterial walls [248, 249]. PPARgamma ligands could not only attenuate the development of PH but could also reverse established pulmonary vascular remodeling.PPARgamma ligands enhanced endothelial nitric oxide production through posttranslational mechanisms that increased nitric oxide synthase activity. Furthermore, PPARgamma ligands inhibited endothelial nicotin amideadenine dinucleotide phosphate (NADPH) oxidaseexpression, activity, and superoxide production. These findings suggest that PPARgamma ligands could restore redox balance in pulmonary circulation to improve endothelial dysfunction, a critical derangement leading to pulmonary vasoconstriction and vascular remodeling [250-253]. Rosiglitazone and pioglitazone are antidiabetic drugs used to control high blood sugar in patients with type 2 diabetes. Side effects of both include heart failure, ischemic cardiovascular risk, fractures, anemia, macular edema, and cancer [254].

Elastase Inhibitors

Administration of elastase inhibitors reverses fatal PH inrats by inducing SMC apoptosis. In pulmonary artery organculture, the mechanism by which elastase inhibitors induce SMC apoptosis involves repression of matrix metalloproteinase activity and subsequent signaling through alphavbeta3-integrins and epidermal growth factor receptors (EGFRs). This suggests that blockade of these downstream effectors may also induce regression of PH. Selective blockade of EGFR signaling may be a novel strategy toreverse progressive, fatal PH [255].

Table 4. Speculative therapeutic options for pulmonary hypertension

Drug	Administration	Administration	Adverse effects
Fasudil	IV	30 mg for 30 min	Flushing
Imatinib	Oral	200 mg qd	Cardiotoxicity
Simvastatin	Oral	20–80 mg qd	Myalgias
Ghrelin		ND	
Bradykinin		ND	
Fluoxetine	Oral	ND	Mild gastrointestinal symptoms
Dichloroacetate	Oral	ND	
Vasoactive intestinal peptide	Inhalation	ND	NA

IV, intravenous; NA, not available; ND, no data; PDEI, phosphodiesterase type 5 inhibitor; PDGF, platelet-derived growth factor; PH, pulmonary hypertension; qd, once daily.

Survivin

Survivin belongs to the family of genes known as inhibitors of apoptosis, and it has been implicated in both prevention of cell death and control of mitosis. McMurtry et al. reported that adenovirus-mediated overexpression of surviving induces PH in rats, whereas inhalation of an adenovirus vector encoding a mutant survivin gene with dominant-negative properties reverses established monocrotaline-induced PH. These findings raise importantissues about the role of survivin in the pathogenesis of PH, its value as a prognostic indicator, and its use as atarget for new therapeutic strategies [256]. The use of molecular antagonists of survivin to increase cell death and to prevent pathological vascular remodeling might hold therapeutic potential [257, 258]

Conclusion

Pulmonary hypertension refers to a clinical syndrome of vascular disease with a stereotyped pattern of histopathology and is related to a variety of secondary disease states. It has become increasingly clear that development of PH entails acomplex, multifactorial pathophysiology. With the availability of multiple agents and the potential for combination therapy, as well as the use of emerging therapies to modify the disease early in its course, the treatment of PH is now entering a new era.

References

[1] Wolter JM, Katrien G. Histopathology of pulmonary hypertensive diseases. *Current Diagnostic Pathology* 2006; 12:429–440.
[2] Chin KM, Kim NH, Rubin LJ.The right ventricle in pulmonary hypertension. *Coron Artery Dis* 2005;16: 13–18.
[3] Stepulmonary hypertensionen YC, Josepulmonary hypertension L. Pathogenic mechanisms of pulmonary hypertension. *Journal of Molecular and Cellular Cardiology* 2008;44:14–30.
[4] Galiè N, Torbicki A, Barst R, et al. Task Force. Task Force Guidelines on diagnosis and treatment of pulmonary hypertension: the task force on diagnosis and treatment of pulmonary hypertension of the European Society of Cardiology. *Eur Heart J* 2004; 25: 2243–2278.
[5] Simonneau G, Robbins IM, Beghetti M, et al. Updated clinical classification of pulmonary hypertension. *J Am Coll Cardiol*. 2009; 54(1 Suppl):S43-54.
[6] Humbert M, Morrell N, Archer S, et al. Cellular and molecular pathobiology of Pulmonary hypertension. *J Am Coll Cardiol* 2004;43(12 Suppl S):13S–24S.

[7] Cool C, Stewart J, Werahera P, et al. Three-dimensional reconstruction of pulmonary arteries in plexiform pulmonary hypertension using cell-specific markers. Evidence for a dynamic and heterogeneous process of pulmonary endothelial cell growth. *Am J Pathol* 1999;155:411–9.

[8] Zhu P, Huang L, Ge X, et al. Transdifferentiation of pulmonary arteriolar endothelial cells into smooth muscle-like cells regulated by myocardin involved in hypoxia-induced pulmonary vascular remodelling. *Int J Exp Pathol* 2006;87:463–74.

[9] Lee S, Shroyer K, Markham N, et al.Monoclonal endothelial cell proliferation is present in primary but not secondary pulmonary hypertension. *J Clin Invest* 1998;101:927–34.

[10] Yeager M, Halley G, Golpon H, et al. Microsatellite instability of endothelial cell growth and apoptosis genes within plexiform lesions in primary pulmonary hypertension. *Circ Res* 2001;88:E2–E11.

[11] Trembath R, Thomson J, Machado R, et al.Clinical and molecular genetic features of pulmonary hypertension in patients with hereditary hemorrhagic telangiectasia. *N Engl J Med* 2001;345:325–34.

[12] Chaouat A, Coulet F, Favre C, et al. Endoglin germline mutation in a patient with hereditary haemorrhagic telangiectasia and dexfenfluramine associated pulmonary hypertension. *Thorax* 2004;59:446–8.

[13] Lane K, Machado R, Pauciulo M, et al.Heterozygous germline mutations in BMPR2, encoding a TGF-beta receptor, cause familial primary pulmonary hypertension. The International PPH Consortium. *Nat Gen* 2000;26:81–4.

[14] Newman J, Wheeler L, Lane K, et al. Mutation in the gene for bone morpulmonary hypertensionogenetic protein receptor II as a cause of primary pulmonary hypertension in a large kindred. *N Engl J Med* 2001;345:319–24.

[15] Aldred M, Machado R, James V, et al. Characterization of the BMPR2 5'-untranslated region and a novel mutation in pulmonary hypertension. *Am J Respir Crit Care Med* 2007;176:819–24.

[16] Sweeney M, Yuan J. Hypoxic pulmonary vasoconstriction: role of voltage-gated potassium channels. *Respir Res* 2000;1:40–8.

[17] Grisaru D, Rachmilewitz E,Mosseri M, et al.Cardiopulmonary assessment in beta-thalassemia major. *Chest* 1990;98:1138–42.

[18] Koren A, Garty I, Antonelli D, et al.Right ventricular cardiac dysfunction in beta-thalassemia major. *Am J Dis Child* 141:93–96.

[19] Minter K, Gladwin M. Pulmonary complications of sickle cell anemia. A need for increased recognition, treatment, and research. *Am J Respir Crit Care Med* 2001;164:2016–9.

[20] Castro O, Hoque M, Brown B. Pulmonary hypertensionin sickle celldisease: cardiac catheterization results and survival. *Blood* 2003;101:1257–61.

[21] Gladwin M, Sachdev V, Jison M, et al. Pulmonary hypertensionas a risk factor for death in patients with sickle cell disease. *N Engl J Med* 2004;350:886–95.

[22] Reiter C, Wang X, Tanus-Santos J, et al. Cell-free hemoglobin limits nitric oxide bioavailability in sickle-cell disease. *Nat Med* 2002;8:1383–9.

[23] Klings E, Farber H. Role of free radicals in the pathogenesis of acute chest syndrome in sickle cell disease. *Respir Res* 2001;2:280–5.

[24] Aslan M, Ryan T, Adler B, et al. Oxygen radical inhibition of nitric oxide-dependent vascular function in sickle cell disease. *Proc Natl Acad Sci U S A* 2001;98:15215–20.

[25] Silver R. Scleroderma. Clinical problems. *The lungs. Rheum Dis Clin North Am* 1996;22:825–40.

[26] Bolster M, Silver R. Lung disease in systemic sclerosis (scleroderma). *Baillière's Clin Rheumatol* 1993;7:79–97.

[27] Battle R, Davitt MCSM, et al. Prevalence of pulmonary hypertension in limited and diffuse scleroderma. *Chest* 1996;110:1515–9.

[28] Ortiz L, Champion H, Lasky J, et al. Enalapril protects mice from pulmonary hypertension by inhibiting TNF mediated activation of NF-kappaB and AP-1. *Am J Pulmonary hypertensionysiol Lung Cell Mol Pulmonary hypertensionysiol* 2002;282:L1209–21.

[29] Speich R, Jenni R, Opravil M, et al. Primary pulmonary hypertension in HIV infection. *Chest* 1991;100:1268–71.

[30] Farber H. HIV-associated pulmonary hypertension. *AIDS Clin Care* 2001;13:53–5.

[31] Galiè N, Manes A, Uguccioni L, et al. Primary pulmonary hypertension: insights into pathogenesis from epidemiology. *Chest* 1998;114(3 Suppl):184S–94S.

[32] Cool C, Kennedy D, Voelkel N, et al. Pathogenesis and evolution of plexiform lesions in pulmonary hypertension associated with scleroderma and human immunodeficiency virus infection. *Human Pathol* 1997;28:434–42.

[33] Kanmogne G., Primeaux C, Grammas P. Induction of apoptosis and endothelin-1 secretion in primary human lung endothelial cells by HIV-1 gp120 proteins. *Biochem Biopulmonary hypertensionys Res Comm* 2005;333(4):333 (334):1107–1115.

[34] Marecki J, Cool C, Parr J, et al.HIV-1 Nef is associated with complex pulmonary vascular lesions in SHIV-nefinfected macaques. *Am J Respir Crit Care Med* 2006;174:437–45.

[35] Steele P, Fuster V, Cohen M, et al. Isolated atrial septal defect with pulmonary vascular obstructive disease-long-term follow-up and prediction of outcome after surgical correction. *Circulation* 1987;76:1037–42.

[36] Topper J, Gimbrone MJ. Blood flow and vascular gene expression: fluid shear stress as a modulator of endothelial pulmonary hypertensionenotype. *Mol Med Today* 1999;5:40–6.

[37] Sakao S, Taraseviciene-Stewart L, Lee J, et al. Initial apoptosis is followed by increased proliferation of apoptosis resistant endothelial cells. *FASEB J* 2005;19:1178–80.

[38] McQuillan L, Leung G, Marsden P, et al. Hypoxia inhibits expression of eNOS via transcriptional and posttranscriptional mechanisms. *Am J Pulmonary hypertensionysiol* 1994;267:H1921–7.

[39] Giaid A, Saleh D. Reduced expression of endothelial nitric oxide ynthase in the lungs of patients with pulmonary hypertension. *N Engl J Med* 1995;333:214–21.

[40] FaganK, Fouty B, Tyler R, et al. The pulmonary circulation of homozygous or heterozygous eNOS-null mice is hyperresponsive tomild hypoxia. *J Clin Invest* 1999;103: 291–9.

[41] Champion H, Bivalacqua T, Greenberg S, et al.Adenoviral gene transfer of endothelial nitric-oxide synthase (eNOS) partially restores normal pulmonary arterial pressure in eNOS-deficient mice. *Proc Natl Acad Sci U S A* 2002;99:13248–53.

[42] Griffiths M, Evans T. Inhaled nitric oxide therapy in adults. *N Engl J Med* 2005;353:2683–95.

[43] Galiè N, Ghofrani H, Torbicki A, et al. Sildenafil citrate therapy for pulmonary hypertension. *N Engl J Med* 2005;353:2148–57.

[44] Barnett C, Machado R. Sildenafil in the treatment of pulmonary hypertension.*VascHealth Risk Manag* 2006;2:411–22.

[45] Yet S, PerrellaM, LayneM, et al. Hypoxia induces severe right ventricular dilatation and infarction in heme oxygenase-1 null mice. *J Clin Invest* 1999;103:R23–9.

[46] Christou H, Morita T, Hsieh C, et al.Prevention of hypoxia-induced pulmonary hypertension by enhancement of endogenous heme oxygenase-1 in the rat. *Circ Res* 2000;86:1224–9.
[47] Zuckerbraun B, Chin B, Wegiel B, et al. Carbon monoxide reverses established pulmonary hypertension. *J Exp Med* 2006;203:2109–19.
[48] Chunyu Z, Junbao D, Dingfang B, et al. The regulatory effect of hydrogen sulfide on hypoxic pulmonary hypertension in rats. Biochem Biopulmonary hypertensionys *Res Commun* 2003;302:810–6.
[49] Li X, Du J, Ding Y, et al.Impact of hydrogen sulfide donor on experimental pulmonary hypertension induced by high pulmonary flow and endogenous carbon monoxide/heme oxygenase pathway. *J Peking Univ Health Sci* 2006;38:135–9
[50] Gerber J, Voelkel N, Nies A, et al. Moderation of hypoxic vasoconstriction by infused arachidonic acid: role of PGI2. *J Appl Physiol* 1980;49:107–12.
[51] Tuder R, Cool C, Geraci M, et al. Prostacyclin synthase expression is decreased in lungs from patients with severe pulmonary hypertension. *Am J Respir Crit Care Med* 1999;159:1925–32.
[52] Christman B, Mc PH C, Newman J, et al. An imbalance between the excretion of thromboxane and prostacyclin metabolites in pulmonary hypertension. *N Engl J Med* 1992;327:70–5.
[53] Strauss W, Edelman J. Prostanoid therapy for pulmonary arterial hypertension. *Clin Chest Med* 2007;28:127–42.
[54] Hassoun P, Thappa V, Landman M, et al. Endothelin 1 mitogenic activity on pulmonary artery smooth muscle cells and release from hypoxic endothelial cells. *Proc Soc Exp Biol Med Soc Exp Biol Med* 1992;199:165–70.
[55] Stelzner T, O'Brien R, Yanagisawa M, et al.Increased lung endothelin-1 production in rats with idiopathic pulmonary hypertension. *Am J Pulmonary hypertensionysiol* 1992;262:L614–20.
[56] Allen S, Chatfield B, Koppenhafer S, et al.Circulating immunoreactive endothelin-1 in children with pulmonary hypertension. Association with acute hypoxic pulmonary vasoreactivity. *Am Rev Respir Dis* 1993;148:519–22.
[57] Giaid A, YanagisawaM, Langleben D, et al. Expression of endothelin-1 in the lungs of patients with pulmonary hypertension. *N Engl J Med* 1993;328:1732–9.
[58] Langleben D. Endothelin receptor antagonists in the treatment of pulmonary arterial hypertension. *Clin Chest Med* 2007;28:117–25.

[59] Cox C, Linden J, Said S. VIP elevates platelet cyclic AMP (cAMP) levels and inhibits in vitro platelet activation induced by platelet-activating factor (PAF). *Peptides* 1984;5:325–8.
[60] Maruno K, Absood A, Said S. VIP inhibits basal and histamine stimulated proliferation of human airway smooth muscle cells. *Am J Pulmonary hypertensionysiol* 1995;268:L1047–51.
[61] PetkovV, MosgoellerW, Ziesche R, et al. Vasoactive intestinal peptide as a new drug for treatment of primary pulmonary hypertension. *J Clin Invest* 2003;111:1339–46.
[62] Caldwell R, Gadipatti R, Lane K, Shepulmonary hypertensionerd V. HIV-1 TAT represses transcription of the bone morpulmonary hypertensionogenic protein receptor-2 in U937 monocytic cells. *J Leukoc Biol* 2006;79:192–201.
[63] Said S, Hamidi S, Dickman K, et al. Moderate pulmonary arterial hypertension in male mice lacking the vasoactive intestinal peptide gene. *Circulation* 2007;115:1260–8.
[64] Söderman C, Eriksson L, Juhlin-Dannfelt A, et al. Effect of vasoactive intestinal polypeptide (VIP) on pulmonary ventilation–perfusion relationships and central haemodynamics in healthy subjects. *Clin Pulmonary hypertensionysiol* 1993;13:677–85.
[65] Gunaydin S, Imai Y, Takanashi Y, et al.The effects of vasoactive intestinal peptide on monocrotaline induced pulmonary hypertensive rabbits following cardiopulmonary bypass: a comparative study with isoproteronol and nitroglycerine. *Cardiovasc Surg* 2002;10:138–45.
[66] Tuder R, Flook B, Voelkel N. Increased gene expression for VEGF and the VEGF receptors KDR/Flk and Flt in lungs exposed to acute or to chronic hypoxia. Modulation of gene expression by nitric oxide. *J Clin Invest* 1995;95:1798–807.
[67] Tuder R, Chacon M, Alger L, et al. Expression of angiogenesis-related molecules in plexiform lesions in severe pulmonary hypertension: evidence for a process of disordered angiogenesis. *J Pathol* 2001;195:367–74.
[68] Wanstall J, Gambino A, Jeffery T, et al. Vascular endothelial growth factor-B-deficient mice show impaired development of hypoxic pulmonary hypertension. *Cardiovasc Res* 2002;55:361–8.
[69] Taraseviciene-Stewart L, Kasahara Y, Alger L, et al. Inhibition of the VEGF receptor 2 combined with chronic hypoxia causes cell death-dependent pulmonary endothelial cell proliferation and severe pulmonary hypertension. *FASEB J* 2001;15: 427–38.

[70] Hansmann G, Wagner R, Schellong S, et al.Pulmonary arterial hypertension is linked to insulin resistance and reversed by peroxisome proliferator-activated receptor-gamma activation. *Circulation* 2007;115:1275–84.
[71] Schermuly R, Pullamsetti S, Kwapiszewska G, et al.Phosphodiesterase 1 upregulation in pulmonary arterial hypertension: target for reverse-remodeling therapy.*Circulation* 2007;115:2331–9.
[72] McMurtry M, Archer S, Altieri D, et al. Gene therapy targeting survivin selectively induces pulmonary vascular apoptosis and reverses pulmonary arterial hypertension. *J Clin Invest* 2005;115:1479–91.
[73] Greenway S, van Suylen R, Du Marchie Sarvaas G, et al. S100A4/Mts1 produces murine pulmonary artery changes resembling plexogenic arteriopathy and is increased in human plexogenic arteriopathy. *Am J Pathol* 2004;164:253–62.
[74] Merklinger S, Wagner R, Spiekerkoetter E, et al.Increased fibulin-5 and elastin in S100A4/Mts1 mice with pulmonary hypertension. *Circ Res* 2005;97:596–604.
[75] YuY, Fantozzi I, Remillard C, et al. Enhanced expression of transient receptor potential channels in idiopathic pulmonary arterial hypertension. *Proc Natl Acad Sci U S A* 2004;101:13861–6.
[76] Shimokubo T, Sakata J, Kitamura K, et al. Augmented adrenomedullin concentrations in right ventricle and plasma of experimental pulmonary hypertension. *Life Sci* 1995;57:1771–9.
[77] Nishikimi T, Nagata S, Sasaki T, et al. Plasma concentrations of adrenomedullin correlate with the extent of pulmonary hypertension in patients with mitral stenosis. *Heart* 1997;78:390–5.
[78] Kakishita M, Nishikimi T, Okano Y, et al.Increased plasma levels of adrenomedullin in patients with pulmonary hypertension. *Clin Sci* 1999;96:33–9.
[79] Loscalzo J, Kohane I, Barabasi A. Human disease classification in the postgenomic era: a complex systems approach to human pathobiology. *Molec Syst Biol* 2007;3:124.
[80] Shimokawa H, Takeshita A. Rho-kinase is an important therapeutic target in cardiovascular medicine. *Arterioscler Thromb Vasc Biol* 2005;25: 1767–75.

[81] Weigand L, Sylvester J, Shimoda L. Mechanisms of endothelin-1-induced contraction in pulmonary arteries from chronically hypoxic rats.*Am J Pulmonary hypertensionysiol Lung Cell Mol Pulmonary hypertensionysiol* 2006;290:L284–90.
[82] Barman S. Vasoconstrictor effect of endothelin-1 on hypertensive pulmonary arterial smooth muscle involves Rho kinase and protein kinase C. *Am J Pulmonary hypertensionysiol Lung Cell Mol Pulmonary hypertensionysiol* 2007;293:L472–9.
[83] Liu Y, Suzuki Y, Day R, et al.Rho kinase-induced nuclear translocation of ERK1/ERK2 in smooth muscle cell mitogenesis caused by serotonin. *Circ Res* 2004;95:579–86.
[84] Li M, Liu Y, Dutt P, Fanburg B, et al. Inhibition of serotonin-induced mitogenesis, migration, and ERK MAPK nuclear translocation in vascular smooth muscle cells by atorvastatin. *Am J Pulmonary hypertensionysiol Lung Cell Mol Pulmonary hypertensionysiol* 2007;293:L463–71.
[85] Takemoto M, Sun J, Hiroki J, et al.Rho-kinase mediates hypoxia-induced downregulation of endothelial nitric oxide synthase. *Circulation* 2002;106:57–62.
[86] Nagaoka T, Morio Y, Casanova N, et al. Rho/Rho kinase signaling mediates increased basal pulmonary vascular tone in chronically hypoxic rats. *Am J Pulmonary hypertensionysiol Lung Cell Mol Pulmonary hypertensionysiol* 2004;287:L665–72.
[87] Oka M, Homma N, Taraseviciene-Stewart L, et al. Rho kinase-mediated vasoconstriction is important in severe occlusive pulmonary arterial hypertension in rats. *Circ Res* 2007;100:923–9.
[88] Fagan K, Oka M, Bauer N, et al. Attenuation of acute hypoxic pulmonary vasoconstriction and hypoxic pulmonary hypertension in mice by inhibition of Rho-kinase. *Am J Pulmonary hypertensionysiol Lung Cell Mol Pulmonary hypertensionysiol* 2004;287:L656–64.
[89] Abe K, Shimokawa H, Morikawa K, et al.Long-term treatment with a Rho-kinase inhibitor improves monocrotaline-induced fatal pulmonary hypertension in rats. *Circ Res* 2004;94:385–93.
[90] Abe K, Tawara S, Oi K, et al. Longterm inhibition of Rho-kinase ameliorates hypoxia-induced pulmonary hypertension in mice. *J Cardiovasc Pulmonary hypertensionarmacol* 2006;48:280–5.
[91] Jiang B, Tawara S, Abe K, et al. Acute vasodilator effect of fasudil, a Rho-kinase inhibitor, in monocrotaline-induced pulmonary hypertension in rats. *J Cardiovasc Pulmonary hypertensionarmacol* 2007;49:85–9.

[92] Li F, XiaW, Li A, et al. Inhibition of rho kinase attenuates high flow induced pulmonary hypertension in rats. *Chin Med J* 2007;120:22–9.
[93] Li F, Xia W, Li A, et al. Long-term inhibition of Rho kinase with fasudil attenuates high flow induced pulmonary artery remodeling in rats. *Pulmonary hypertensionarmacol Res* 2007;55:64–71.
[94] Fukumoto Y, Matoba T, Ito A, et al. Acute vasodilator effects of a Rho-kinase inhibitor, fasudil, in patients with severe pulmonary hypertension. *Heart* 2005;91:391–2.
[95] Ishikura K, Yamada N, Ito M, et al.Beneficial acute effects of rho-kinase inhibitor in patients with pulmonary arterial hypertension. *Circ J* 2006;70:174–8.
[96] Nishimura T, Faul J, Berry G, et al.Simvastatin attenuates smooth muscle neointimal proliferation and pulmonary hypertension in rats. *Am J Respir Crit Care Med* 2002;166:1403–8.
[97] Hu H, Sung A, Zhao G, et al. Simvastatin enhances bonemorpulmonary hypertensionogenetic protein receptor type II expression. *Biochem Biopulmonary hypertensionys Res Commun 2006*;339:59–64.
[98] Moudgil R, Michelakis E, Archer S. The role of K+ channels in determining pulmonary vascular tone, oxygen sensing, cell proliferation, and apoptosis: implications in hypoxic pulmonary vasoconstriction and pulmonary arterial hypertension. *Microcirculation* 2006;13:615–32.
[99] Yuan X,Wang J, Juhaszova M, et al. Attenuated K+ channel gene transcription in primary pulmonary hypertension. *Lancet* 1998;351: 726–7.
[100] Remillard C, Tigno D, Platoshyn O, et al. Function of Kv1.5 channels and genetic variations of KCNA5 in patients with idiopathic pulmonary arterial hypertension. *Am J Pulmonary hypertensionysiol Cell Pulmonary hypertensionysiol* 2007;292:C1837–53.
[101] Weir E, Reeve H, Huang J, et al. Anorexic agents aminorex, fenfluramine, and dexfenfluramine inhibit potassium current in rat pulmonary vascular smooth muscle and cause pulmonary vasoconstriction. *Circulation* 1996;94:2216–20.
[102] Cogolludo A, Moreno L, Lodi F, et al.Serotonin inhibits voltage-gated K+ currents in pulmonary artery smooth muscle cells: role of 5-HT2A receptors, caveolin-1, and KV1.5 channel internalization. *Circ Res* 2006;98:931–8.
[103] Cogolludo A, Moreno L, Bosca L, et al.Thromboxane A2-induced inhibition of voltage-gated K+ channels and pulmonary vasoconstriction: role of protein kinase Czeta. *Circ Res* 2003;93:656–63.

[104] Michelakis E, McMurtryM, Sonnenberg B, et al. The NO-K+ channel axis in pulmonary arterial hypertension. Activation by experimental oral therapies. *Adv Exp Med Biol* 2003;543:293-322.
[105] Young K, Ivester C, West J, et al.BMP signaling controls PASMC KV channel expression in vitro and in vivo. *Am J Pulmonary hypertensionysiol Lung Cell Mol Pulmonary hypertensionysiol* 2006;290:L841-8.
[106] Fantozzi I, Platoshyn O,Wong A, et al. Bone morpulmonary hypertension-ogenetic protein-2 upregulates expression and function of voltage-gated K+ channels in human pulmonary artery smooth muscle cells. *Am J Pulmonary hypertensionysiol Lung Cell Mol Pulmonary hypertensionysiol* 2006;291:L993-L1004.
[107] Pozeg Z, Michelakis E, McMurtry M, et al. In vivo gene transfer of the O2-sensitive potassium channel Kv1.5 reduces pulmonary hypertension and restores hypoxic pulmonary vasoconstriction in chronically hypoxic rats. *Circulation* 2003;107:2037-44.
[108] BrindleN, Saharinen P,AlitaloK. Signaling and functions of angiopoietin-1 in vascular protection. *Circ Res* 2006;98:1014-23.
[109] Kugathasan L, Dutly A, Zhao Y, et al.Role of angiopoietin-1 in experimental and human pulmonary arterial hypertension. *Chest* 2005;128(6 Suppl):633S-42S.
[110] Dewachter L,Adnot S, Fadel E, et al.Angiopoietin/Tie2 pathway influences smooth muscle hyperplasia in idiopathic pulmonary hypertension. *Am J Respir Crit Care Med* 2006;1743:1025-33.
[111] Kido M, Du L, Sullivan C, et al. Gene transfer of a TIE2 receptor antagonist prevents pulmonary hypertension in rodents. *J Thorac Cardiovasc Surg* 2005;129:268-76.
[112] EickelbergO,Yeager M,Grimminger F. The tantalizing triplet of pulmonary hypertension-BMP receptors, serotonin receptors, and angiopoietins. *Cardiovasc Res* 2003;60:465-7.
[113] Zhao Y, Campbell A, Robb M, et al.Protective role of angiopoietin-1 in experimental pulmonary hypertension. *Circ Res* 2003;92:984-91.
[114] Li X, Everson W, Smart E. Caveolae, lipid rafts, and vascular disease. *Trends Cardiovasc Med* 2005;15:92-6.
[115] Zhao Y, Liu Y, Stan R, et al.Defects in caveolin-1 cause dilated cardiomyopathy and pulmonary hypertension in knockout mice. *Proc Natl Acad Sci U S A* 2002;99:11375-80.

[116] Drab M, Verkade P, Elger M, et al. Loss of caveolae, vascular dysfunction, and pulmonary defects in caveolin-1 gene-disrupted mice. *Science* 2001;293:2449–52.
[117] Shaul P, Smart E, Robinson L, et al. Acylation targets endothelial nitric-oxide synthase to plasmalemmal caveolae. *J Biol Chem* 1996;271:6518–22.
[118] Chun M, Liyanage U, Lisanti M, et al. Signal transduction of a G protein-coupled receptor in caveolae: colocalization of endothelin and its receptor with caveolin. *Proc Natl Acad Sci U S A* 1994;91:11728–32.
[119] Sehgal P, Mukhopadhyay S, Xu F, et al. Dysfunction of Golgi tethers, SNAREs, and SNAPs in monocrotaline-induced pulmonary hypertension. *Am J Pulmonary hypertensionysiol Lung Cell Mol Pulmonary hypertensionysiol* 2007;292:L1526–42.
[120] Ramos M, Lamé M, Segall H, et al. The BMP type II receptor is located in lipid rafts, including caveolae, of pulmonary endothelium in vivo and in vitro. *Vasc Pulmonary hypertensionarmacol* 2006;44:50–9.
[121] Wiechen K, Sers C, Agoulnik A, et al. Downregulation of caveolin-1, a candidate tumor suppressor gene, in sarcomas. *Am J Pathol* 2001;158:833–9.
[122] Gillespie M, Goldblum S, Cohen D, et al.Interleukin 1 bioactivity in the lungs of rats with monocrotaline-induced pulmonary hypertension. *Proc Soc Exp Biol Med* 1988;187:26–32.
[123] Perkett E, Lyons R, Moses H, et al.Transforming growth factor-beta activity in sheep lung lympulmonary hypertension during the development of pulmonary hypertension. *J Clin Invest* 1990;86:1459–64.
[124] Chand N, Altura B. Acetylcholine and bradykinin relax intrapulmonary arteries by acting on endothelial cells: role in lung vascular diseases. *Science* 1981;213:1376–9.
[125] Itoh T, Nagaya N, Ishibashi-Ueda H, et al. Increased plasma monocyte chemoattractant protein-1 level in idiopathic pulmonary arterial hypertension. *Respirol* 2006;11:158–63.
[126] Balabanian K, Foussat A, Dorfmüller P, et al. CX(3)C chemokine fractalkine in pulmonary arterial hypertension. *Am J Respir Crit Care Med* 2002;165:1419–25.
[127] Dorfmüller P, Zarka V, Durand-Gasselin I, et al.Chemokine RANTES in severe pulmonary arterial hypertension. *Am J Respir Crit Care Med* 2002;165:534–9.

[128] Stenmark K, James S, Voelkel N, et al. Leukotriene C4 and D4 in neonates with hypoxemia and pulmonary hypertension. *N Engl J Med* 1983;309:77–80.
[129] Voelkel N, Tuder R, Wade K, et al. Inhibition of 5-lipoxygenase-activating protein (FLAP) reduces pulmonary vascular reactivity and pulmonary hypertension in hypoxic rats. *J Clin Invest* 1996;97:2491–8.
[130] Wright L, Tuder R,Wang J, et al. 5-Lipoxygenase and 5-lipoxygenase activating protein (FLAP) immunoreactivity in lungs from patients with primary pulmonary hypertension. *Am J Respir Crit Care Med* 1998;157:219–29.
[131] Jones J, Walker J, Song Y, et al. Effect of 5-lipoxygenase on the development of pulmonary hypertension in rats. Am J Pulmonary hypertensionysiol *Heart Circ Pulmonary hypertensionysiol* 2004;286:H1775–84.
[132] Rabinovitch M. Pathobiology of pulmonary hypertension. Extracellular matrix. *Clin Chest Med* 2001;22:433–49.
[133] Rabinovitch M. Elastase and the pathobiology of unexplained pulmonary hypertension. *Chest* 1998;114(3 Suppl):213S–24S.
[134] Zhu L, Wigle D, Hinek A, et al. The endogenous vascular elastase that governs development and progression of monocrotaline-induced pulmonary hypertension in rats is a novel enzyme related to the serine proteinase adipsin. *J Clin Invest* 1994;94:1163–71.
[135] Jones P, Rabinovitch M. Tenascin-C is induced with progressive pulmonary vascular disease in rats and is functionally related to increased smooth muscle cell proliferation. *Circ Res* 1996;79:1131–42.
[136] Ihida-Stansbury K, McKean D, Lane K, et al. Tenascin-C is induced by mutated BMP type II receptors in familial forms of pulmonary arterial hypertension. *Am J Pulmonary hypertensionysiol Lung Cell Mol Pulmonary hypertensionysiol* 2006;291:L694–702.
[137] Mitani Y, Zaidi S, Dufourcq P, et al.Nitric oxide reduces vascular smooth muscle cell elastase activity through cGMP mediated suppression of ERK pulmonary hypertensionospulmonary hypertensionorylation and AML1B nuclear partitioning. *FASEB J* 2000;14:805–14.
[138] Cowan K, Jones P, RabinovitchM. Elastase and matrix metalloproteinase inhibitors induce regression, and tenascin-C antisense prevents progression, of vascular disease. *J Clin Invest* 2000;105:21–34.

[139] Cowan K, Heilbut A, Humpl T, et al.Complete reversal of fatal pulmonary hypertension in rats by a serine elastase inhibitor. *Nat Med* 2000;6:698–702.
[140] Launay J, Hervé P, Peoc'h KTC, et al.Function of the serotonin 5-hydroxytryptamine 2B receptor in pulmonary hypertension. *Nat Med* 2002;8:1129–35.
[141] Zaidi S, You X, Ciura S, et al.Overexpression of the serine elastase inhibitor elafin protects transgenic mice from hypoxic pulmonary hypertension. *Circulation* 2002;105:516–21,
[142] S.A. van Wolferen, K. Gru"nberg, A. Vonk Noordegraaf,Diagnosis and management of pulmonary hypertension over the past 100 years. *Respiratory Medicine* 2007; 101:389–398
[143] Puri A, McGoon MD, Kushwaha SS. Pulmonary hypertension: current therapeutic strategies.*Nat Clin Pract Cardiovasc Med.* 2007;4:319-29.
[144] Ahearn GS, Tapson VF, Rebeiz A, et al. Electrocardiograpulmonary hypertensiony to define clinical status in primary pulmonary hypertension and pulmonary hypertension secondary to collagen vascular disease. *Chest.* 2002;122:524-7.
[145] Karazincir S, Balci A, Seyfeli E, et al. CT assessment of main pulmonary artery diameter. *Diagn Interv Radiol.* 2008;14:72-4.
[146] Edwards PD, Bull RK, Coulden R. CT measurement of main pulmonary artery diameter. *Br J Radiol.* 1998;71:1018-20.
[147] Fisher MR, Forfia PR, Chamera E, et al.Accuracy of Doppler echocardiograpulmonary hypertensiony in the hemodynamic assessment of pulmonary hypertension. *Am J Respir Crit Care Med.* 2009;179:615-21.
[148] Forfia PR, Fisher MR, Mathai SC, et al.Tricuspid annular displacement predicts survival in pulmonary hypertension. *Am J Respir Crit Care Med.* 2006;174:1034-41.
[149] Steendijk P. Right ventricular function and failure: methods, models, and mechanisms. *Crit Care Med.* 2004;32:1087-9.
[150] Woods J, Monteiro P, Rhodes A. Right ventricular dysfunction. *Curr Opin Crit Care.* 2007;13:532-40.
[151] Kosiborod M, Wackers FJ. Assessment of right ventricular morpulmonary hypertensionology and function. *Semin Respir Crit Care Med.* 2003;24:245-62.

[152] Marcus JT, Vonk Noordegraaf A, Roeleveld RJ, et al.Impaired left ventricular filling due to right ventricular pressure overload in primary pulmonary hypertension: noninvasive monitoring using MRI. *Chest.* 2001;119:1761-5.
[153] Dellegrottaglie S, Sanz J, Poon M, et al. Pulmonary hypertension: accuracy of detection with left ventricular septal-to-free wall curvature ratio measured at cardiac MR. *Radiology.* 2007;243:63-9.
[154] Gan CT, Lankhaar JW, Westerhof N, et al.Noninvasively assessed pulmonary artery stiffness predicts mortality in Pulmonary hypertension. *Chest.* 2007;132:1906-12.
[155] Jardim C, Rochitte CE, Humbert M, et al. Pulmonary artery distensibility in pulmonary hypertension: an MRI pilot study. *Eur Respir J.* 2007;29:476-81.
[156] Sanz J, Kuschnir P, Rius T, et al. Pulmonary hypertension: noninvasive detection with pulmonary hypertensionase-contrast MR imaging. *Radiology.* 2007;243:70-9.
[157] Chin KM, Kingman M, de Lemos JA, et al. Changes in right ventricular structure and function assessed using cardiac magnetic resonance imaging in bosentan-treated patients with pulmonary hypertension. *Am J Cardiol.* 2008;101:1669-72.
[158] Roeleveld RJ, Vonk-Noordegraaf A, Marcus JT, et al. Effects of epoprostenol on right ventricular hypertropulmonary hypertensiony and dilatation in pulmonary hypertension. *Chest.* 2004;125:572-9.
[159] Reesink HJ, Marcus JT, Tulevski II, et al. Reverse right ventricular remodeling after pulmonary endarterectomy in patients with chronic thromboembolic pulmonary hypertension: utility of magnetic resonance imaging to demonstrate restoration of the right ventricle. *J Thorac Cardiovasc Surg.* 2007;133:58-64.
[160] Sitbon O, Humbert M, Jagot JL, et al. Inhaled nitric oxide as a screening agent for safely identifying responders to oral calcium-channel blockers in primary pulmonary hypertension. *Eur Respir J.* 1998;12:265-70.
[161] Sitbon O, Humbert M, Jaïs X, Ioos V, et al. Long-term response to calcium channel blockers in idiopathic pulmonary hypertension. *Circulation.* 2005;111:3105-11.
[162] Woodmansey PA, O'Toole L, Channer KS, et al.Acute pulmonary vasodilatory properties of amlodipine in humans with pulmonary hypertension. *Heart* 1996; 75: 171–173.

[163] Franz IW, Van Der Meyden J, Schaupp S, et al.The effect of amlodipine on exercise-induced pulmonary hypertension and right heart function in patients with chronic obstructive pulmonary disease. *Z Kardiol* 2002;91: 833–839.
[164] Sitbon O, Humbert M, Jaïs X, et al. Long-term response to calcium channel blockers in idiopathic pulmonary hypertension. *Circulation* 2005; 111: 3105–3111.
[165] Fuster V, Steele PM, Edwards WD, et al. Primary pulmonary hypertension: natural history and the importance of thrombosis. *Circulation* 1984;70: 580–587.
[166] Robbins IM, Kawut SM, Yung D, et al. A study of aspirin and clopidogrel in idiopathic Pulmonary hypertension. *Eur Respir J* 2006; 27: 578–584.
[167] Veyssier-Belot C, Cacoub P. Role of endothelial and smooth muscle cells in the pulmonary hypertensionysiopathology and treatment management of pulmonary hypertension. *Cardiovasc Res* 1999; 44: 274–282.
[168] Barst RJ, Rubin LJ, Long WA, et al.A comparison of continuous intravenous epoprostenol (prostacyclin) with conventional therapy for primary pulmonary hypertension: the Primary pulmonary hypertension Study Group. *N Engl J Med* 1996; 334: 296–302.
[169] McLaughlin VV, Shillington A, Rich S. Survival in primary pulmonary hypertension: the impact of epoprostenol therapy. *Circulation* 2002; 106: 1477–1482.
[170] Sitbon O, Humbert M, Nunes H, et al.Long-term intravenous epoprostenol infusion in primary pulmonary hypertension: prognostic factors and survival. *J AmColl Cardiol* 2002; 40: 780–788.
[171] Simonneau G, Barst RJ, Galie N, et al. Treprostinil Study Group. Continuous subcutaneous infusion of treprostinil, a prostacyclin analogue, in patients with pulmonary hypertension: a double-blind, randomized, placebo-controlled trial. *Am J Respir Crit Care Med* 2002; 165: 800–804.
[172] McLaughlin VV, Gaine SP, Barst RJ, et al.Treprostinil Study Group. Efficacy and safety of treprostinil: an epoprostenol analog for primary pulmonary hypertension. *J Cardiovasc Pulmonary hypertensionarmacol* 2003;41: 293–299.
[173] Gomberg-Maitland M, Tapson VF, Benza RL, et al. Transition from intravenous epoprostenol to intravenous treprostinil in pulmonary hypertension. *Am J Respir Crit Care Med*172: 1586–1589.

[174] Hoeper MM, Olschewski H, Ghofrani HA, et al.A comparison of the acute hemodynamic effects of inhaled nitric oxide and aerosolized iloprost in primary pulmonary hypertension: German PPH study group. *J Am CollCardiol* 2000; 35: 176–182.

[175] Hoeper MM, Schwarze M, Ehlerding S, et al.Long-term treatment of primary pulmonary hypertension with aerosolized iloprost, a prostacyclin analogue. *N Engl J Med* 2000; 342: 1866–1870.

[176] Nagaya N, Uematsu M, Okano Y, et al. Effect of orally active prostacyclin analogue on survival of outpatients with primary pulmonary hypertension. *J Am Coll* Cardiol 1999; 34: 1188–1192.

[177] Galiè N, Humbert M, Vachiéry JL, et al. Arterial Pulmonary Hypertension and Beraprost European (ALPPHABET) Study Group. Arterial pulmonary hypertension and Beraprost European (ALPPHABET) Study Group (2002) Effects of beraprost sodium, an oral prostacyclin analogue, in patients with Pulmonary hypertension: a randomized, double-blind, placebocontrolled trial. *J Am Coll Cardiol* 2002; 39: 1496–1502.

[178] Friesen RH, Williams GD. Anesthetic management of children with pulmonary arterial hypertension. *Pediatric Anesthesia* 2008;18:208-216.

[179] Girard C, Fargnoli JM, Godin-Ribuot D et al. Inhaled nitric oxide: effects on hemodynamics, myocardial contractility, and regional blood flow in dogs with mechanically induced pulmonary artery hypertension. *J Heart Lung Transplant* 1996;15:700–708.

[180] Sitbon O, Humbert M, Jagot JL et al. Inhaled nitric oxide as a screening agent for safely identifying responders to oral calcium-channel blockers in primary pulmonary hypertension. *Eur Respir J* 1998;12:265–270.

[181] Ricciardi MJ, Knight BP, Martinez FJ, et al.Inhaled nitric oxide in primary pulmonary hypertension: a safe and effective agent for predicting response to nifedipine. *J Am Coll Cardiol* 1998;32:1068–1073.

[182] Sitbon O, Brenot F, Denjean A et al. Inhaled nitric oxide as a screening vasodilator agent in primary pulmonary hypertension. A dose-response study and comparison with prostacyclin. *Am J Respir Crit Care Med* 1995;151(2 Pt 1):384–389.

[183] Parsons S, Celermajer D, Savidis E, et al. The effect of inhaled nitric oxide on 6-minute walk distance in patients with pulmonary hypertension. *Chest* 1998;114(1 Suppl):70S–72S.

[184] Galié N, Badesch D, Oudiz R, et al. Ambrisentan therapy for pulmonary hypertension. *J Am Coll Cardiol* 2005; 46: 529–535.

[185] Tantini B, Manes A, Fiumana E, et al. Antiproliferative effect of sildenafil on human pulmonary artery smooth muscle cells. *Basic Res Cardiol* 2005; 100: 131–138.
[186] Prasad S, Wilkinson J, Gatzoulis MA. Sildenafil in primary pulmonary hypertension. *N Engl J Med* 2000; 343: 1342.
[187] Bhatia S, Frantz RP, Severson CJ, et al. Immediate and long-term hemodynamic and clinical effects of sildenafil in patients with pulmonary hypertension receiving vasodilator therapy. *Mayo Clin Proc* 2003; 78: 1207–1213.
[188] Michelakis ED, Tymchak W, Noga M, et al. Long-term treatment with oral sildenafil is safe and improves functional capacity and hemodynamics in patients with pulmonary hypertension. *Circulation* 2003; 108: 2066–2069.
[189] Sastry BK, Narasimhan C, Reddy NK, et al. Clinical efficacy of sildenafil in primary pulmonary hypertension: a randomized, placebo-controlled, double-blind, crossover study. *J Am Coll Cardiol* 2004; 43: 1149–1153.
[190] Galiè N, Ghofrani HA, Torbicki A, et al. Sildenafil Use in Pulmonary Arterial Hypertension (SUPER) Study Group. Sildenafil citrate therapy for pulmonary hypertension. *N Engl J Med* 2005; 353: 2148–2157.
[191] Affuso F, Palmieri EA, Di Conza P, et al. Tadalafil improves quality of life and exercise tolerance in idiopathic pulmonary hypertension. *Int J Cardiol* 2006; 108: 429–431.
[192] Cacoub P, Dorent R, Maistre G, et al. Endothelin-1 in primary pulmonary hypertension and the Eisenmenger syndrome. *Am J Cardiol* 1993; 71: 448–450.
[193] Giaid A, Yanagisawa M, Langleben D, et al. Expression of endothelin-1 in the lungs of patients with pulmonary hypertension. *N Engl J Med* 1993; 328: 1732–1739.
[194] Kedzierski RM, Yanagisawa M. Endothelin system: the double-edged sword in health and disease. *Annu RevPulmonary hypertensionarmacol Toxicol* 2001; 41: 851–876.
[195] Rubin LJ, Badesch DB, Barst RJ, et al.Bosentan therapy for pulmonary hypertension. *N Engl J Med* 2002; 346: 896–903.
[196] Galié N, Manes A, Branzi A. The endothelin system in Pulmonary hypertension. *Cardiovasc Res* 2004; 61: 227–237.
[197] Galié N, Hinderliter AL, Torbicki A, et al. Effects of the oral endothelinreceptor antagonist bosentan on echocardiographic and doppler measures in patients with Pulmonary hypertension. *J Am Coll Cardiol* 2003; 41: 1380–1386.

[198] Channick R, Badesch DB, Tapson VF, et al. Effects of the dual endothelin receptor antagonist bosentan in patients with pulmonary hypertension: a placebo-controlled study. *J Heart Lung Transplant* 2001; 20: 262–263.
[199] Barst RJ, Langleben D, Frost A, et al.STRIDE-1 Study Group. Sitaxsentan therapy for Pulmonary hypertension. *Am J Respir Crit CareMed* 2004; 169: 441–447.
[200] Barst RJ, Langleben D, Badesch D, et al. STRIDE-2 Study Group.Treatment of pulmonary hypertension with the selective endothelin-A receptor antagonist sitaxsentan. *J Am Coll Cardiol* 2006; 47: 2049–2056.
[201] Billman GE. Ambrisentan (Myogen). *Curr Opin Investig Drugs* 2002; 3: 1483–1486.
[202] Humbert M, Barst RJ, Robbins IM, et al. Combination of bosentan with epoprostenol in pulmonary hypertension: BREATHE-2. *Eur Respir J* 2004; 24: 353–359.
[203] Hoeper MM, Leuchte H, Halank M, et al. Combining inhaled iloprost with bosentan in patients with idiopathic pulmonary hypertension. *Eur Respir J* 2006; 28: 691–694.
[204] Seyfarth HJ, Pankau H, Hammerschmidt S, et al. Bosentan improves exercise tolerance and Tei index in patients with pulmonary hypertension and prostanoid therapy. *Chest* 2005; 128: 709–713.
[205] McLaughlin VV, Oudiz RJ, Frost A, et al.Randomized study of adding inhaled iloprost to existing bosentan in pulmonary hypertension. *Am J Respir Crit Care Med* 2006; 174: 1257–1263.
[206] Gomberg-Maitland M. Learning to pair therapies and the expanding matrix for pulmonary hypertension: is more better? *Eur Respir J* 2006; 28: 683–686.
[207] Wilkens H, Guth A, König J, et al. Effect of inhaled iloprost plus oral sildenafil in patients with primary pulmonary hypertension. *Circulation* 2001; 104: 1218–1222.
[208] Gomberg-Maitland M, McLaughlin V, Gulati M, et al. Efficacy and safety of sildenafil added to treprostinil in pulmonary hypertension. *Am J Cardiol* 2005; 96: 1334–1336.
[209] Clozel M, Hess P, Rey M, et al.Bosentan, sildenafil, and their combination in the monocrotaline model of pulmonary hypertension in rats. *Exp Biol Med (Maywood)* 2006; 231: 967–973.
[210] Hoeper MM, Faulenbach C, Golpon H, et al. Combination therapy with bosentan and sildenafil in idiopathic pulmonary hypertension. *Eur Respir J* 2004; 24: 1007–1010.

[211] Morice AH, Mulrennan S, Clark A. Combination therapy with bosentan and pulmonary hypertensionospulmonary hypertensionodiesterase-5 inhibitor in pulmonary hypertension. *Eur Respir J* 2005; 26: 180.
[212] Nazzareno G, Alessandra M, Massimiliano P, et al.Management of pulmonary hypertension associated with congenital systemic-to-pulmonary shunts and Eisenmenger's syndrome. *Drugs* 2008; 68: 1049-1066
[213] Klepetko W, Mayer E, Sandoval J, et al. Interventional and surgical modalities of treatment for pulmonary arterial hypertension. *J Am Coll Cardiol* 2004; 43 (12 Suppl. S): 73-80S
[214] Nagaoka T, Gebb SA, Karoor V, et al. Involvement of RhoA/Rho kinase signaling in pulmonary hypertension of the fawn-hooded rat. *J Appl Physiol* 2006; 100: 996–1002.
[215] Abe K, Shimokawa H, Morikawa K, et al. Long-term treatment with a Rhokinase inhibitor improves monocrotaline-induced fatal pulmonary hypertension in rats. *Circ Res* 2004; 94: 385–393.
[216] Ishikura K, Yamada N, Ito M, et al. Beneficial acute effects of rhokinase inhibitor in patients with pulmonary hypertension. *Circ J* 2006; 70: 174–178.
[217] Guilluy C, Sauzeau V, Rolli-Derkinderen M, et al. Inhibition of RhoA/Rho kinase pathway is involved in the beneficial effect of sildenafil on pulmonary hypertension. *Br J Pulmonary hypertensionarmacol* 2005; 146: 1010–1018.
[218] 65 Barst RJ. PDGF signaling in pulmonary hypertension. *J Clin Invest* 2005; 115: 2691–2694.
[219] Dingli D, Utz JP, Krowka MJ, et al.Unexplained pulmonary hypertension in chronic myeloproliferative disorders. *Chest* 2001; 120: 801–808.
[220] Hoffman R.Is bone marrow fibrosis the real problem? *Blood* 2006; 107: 3421–3422.
[221] Schermuly RT, Dony E, Ghofrani HA, et al. Reversal of experimental pulmonary hypertension by PDGF inhibition. *J ClinInvest* 2005; 115: 2811–2821.
[222] Ghofrani HA, Seeger W, Grimminger F. Imatinib for the treatment of pulmonary hypertension. *N Engl J Med* 2005; 353: 1412–1413.
[223] Souza R, Sitbon O, Parent F, et al.Long term imatinib treatment in pulmonary hypertension. *Thorax* 2006; 61: 736.
[224] Patterson KC, Weissmann A, Ahmadi T, et al. Imatinib mesylate in the treatment of refractory idiopathic pulmonary hypertension. *Ann Intern Med* 2006; 145: 152–153.

[225] Kerkelä R, Grazette L, Yacobi R, et al.Cardiotoxicity of the cancer therapeutic agent imatinib mesylate. *Nat Med* 2006; 12: 908–916.
[226] Hu H, Sung A, Zhao G, et al. Simvastatin enhances bone morpulmonary hypertensionogenetic protein receptor type II expression. Biochem *Biopulmonary hypertensionys Res Commun* 2006; 339: 59–64.
[227] Taraseviciene-Stewart L, Scerbavicius R, Choe KH, et al. Simvastatin causes endothelial cell apoptosis and attenuates severe pulmonary hypertension. *Am J Pulmonary hypertensionysiol LungCell Mol Pulmonary hypertensionysiol* 2006; 291: L668–L676.
[228] Kao PN. Simvastatin treatment of pulmonary hypertension: an observational case series. *Chest* 2005;127: 1446–1452.
[229] Henriques-Coelho T, Roncon-Albuquerque Júnior R, Lourenço AP, et al. Ghrelin reverses molecular, structural and hemodynamic alterations of the right ventricle in pulmonary hypertension. *Rev PortCardiol* 2006; 25: 55–63.
[230] Taraseviciene-Stewart L, Scerbavicius R, Stewart JM, et al. Treatment of severe pulmonary hypertension: a bradykinin receptor 2 agonist B9972 causes reduction of pulmonary artery pressure and right ventricular hypertropulmonary hypertensiony. *Peptides* 2005; 26: 1292–300.
[231] Marcos E, Fadel E, Sanchez O, et al. Serotonin-induced smooth muscle hyperplasia in various forms of human pulmonary hypertension. *Circ Res* 2004; 94: 1263–1270.
[232] golludo A, Moreno L, Lodi F, et al. Serotonin inhibits voltage-gated K+ currents in pulmonary artery smooth muscle cells: role of 5-HT2A receptors, caveolin-1, and Kv1.5 channel internalization. *Circ Res* 2006; 98: 931–938.
[233] Guignabert C, Raffestin B, Benferhat R, et al. Serotonin transporter inhibition prevents and reverses monocrotaline-induced pulmonary hypertension in rats. *Circulation* 2005; 111: 2812–2819.
[234] Petkov V, Gentscheva T, Schamberger C, et al. The vasoactive intestinal peptide receptor turnover in pulmonary arteries indicates an important role for VIP in the rat lung circulation. *AnnNY Acad Sci* 2006; 1070: 481–483.
[235] Petkov V, Mosgoeller W, Ziesche R, et al.Vasoactive intestinal peptide as a new drug for treatment of primary pulmonary hypertension. *J Clin Invest* 2003; 111: 1339–1346.
[236] Guignabert C, Raffestin B, Benferhat R, et al. Serotonin transporter inhibition prevents and reverses monocrotaline-induced pulmonary hypertension in rats.*Circulation* 2005; 111:2812–2819.

[237] Chambers CD, Hernandez-Diaz S, Van Marter LJ, et al. Selective serotoninreuptake inhibitors and risk of persistent pulmonary hypertension of the newborn. *N Engl J Med* 2006; 354:579–587.
[238] Pozeg ZI, Michelakis ED, McMurtry MS, et al. In vivo gene transfer of the O2-sensitive potassium channel Kv1.5 reduces pulmonary hypertension and restores hypoxic pulmonary vasoconstriction in chronically hypoxic rats. *Circulation* 2003; 107:2037–2044.
[239] Reeve HL, Michelakis E, Nelson DP, et al. Alterations in a redox oxygen sensing mechanism in chronic hypoxia. *J Appl Physiol* 2001; 90:2249–2256.
[240] Remillard CV, Yuan JX. Activation of Kt channels: an essential pathway in programmed cell death. *Am J Pulmonary hypertensionysiol Lung Cell Mol Pulmonary hypertensionysiol* 2004; 286:L49–L67.
[241] McMurtry MS, Bonnet S, Wu X, et al. Dichloroacetate prevents and reverses pulmonary hypertension by inducing pulmonary artery smooth muscle cell apoptosis. *Circ Res* 2004; 95:830–840.
[242] Izumi Y, Kim S, Yoshiyama M, et al. Activation of apoptosis signal-regulating kinase 1 in injured artery and its critical role in neointimal hyperplasia. *Circulation* 2003;108:2812–2818.
[243] Hart CM. The role of PPARgamma in pulmonary vascular disease. *J Investig Med* 2008; 56:518–521.
[244] Ameshima S, Golpon H, Cool CD, et al.Peroxisome proliferator-activated receptor gamma (PPARgamma) expression is decreased in pulmonary hypertension and affects endothelial cell growth. *Circ Res* 2003; 92:1162–1169.
[245] Matsuda Y, Hoshikawa Y, Ameshima S, et al.Effects of peroxisome proliferator-activated receptor gamma ligands on monocrotaline-induced pulmonary hypertension in rats. *Nihon Kokyuki Gakkai Zasshi* 2005; 43:283–288.
[246] Crossno JT Jr, Garat CV, Reusch JE, et al.Rosiglitazone attenuates hypoxia-induced pulmonary arterial remodeling. Am J Pulmonary hypertensionysiol. *Am J Physiol Lung Cell Mol Physiol* 2007; 292:L885–L897.
[247] Nisbet R, Kleinhenz D, Thorson H et al. Rosiglitazone attenuates chronic hypoxia-induced pulmonary hypertension. *Am J Respir Crit Care Med* 2007; 175:A43.

[248] Calnek DS, Mazzella L, Roser S, et al.Peroxisome proliferator-activated receptor gamma ligands increase release of nitric oxide from endothelial cells. *Arterioscler Thromb Vasc Biol* 2003; 23:52–57.

[249] Polikandriotis JA, Mazzella LJ, Rupnow HL, et al.Peroxisome proliferator-activated receptor gamma ligands stimulate endothelial nitric oxide production through distinct peroxisome proliferator-activated receptor gamma-dependent mechanisms. *Arterioscler Thromb Vasc Biol* 2005; 25:1810–1816.

[250] Hwang J, Kleinhenz DJ, Lassegue B, et al.Peroxisome proliferator-activated receptorgamma ligands regulate endothelial membrane superoxide production. *Am J Physiol Cell Physiol* 2005; 288:C899–C905.

[251] Hwang J, Kleinhenz DJ, Rupnow HL, et al.The PPAR gamma ligand, rosiglitazone, reduces vascular oxidative stress and NADPH oxidase expression in diabetic mice. *Vascul Pharmacol* 2007; 46:456–462.

[252] Singh S, Loke YK. The safety of rosiglitazone in the treatment of type 2 diabetes. *Expert Opin Drug Saf* 2008; 7:579–585.

[253] Merklinger SL, Jones PL, Martinez EC, et al. Epidermal growth factor receptor blockade mediates smooth muscle cell apoptosis and improves survival in rats with pulmonary hypertension. *Circulation* 2005; 112:423–431.

[254] Blanc-Brude OP, Yu J, Simosa H, et al. Inhibitor of apoptosis protein survivin regulates vascular injury. *Nat Med* 2002; 8:987–994.

[255] Altieri DC. Validating survivin as a cancer therapeutic target. *Nat Rev Cancer* 2003; 3:46–54.

[256] Mita AC, Mita MM, Nawrocki ST, et al.Survivin: key regulator of mitosis and apoptosis and novel target for cancer therapeutics. *Clin Cancer Res* 2008; 14:5000–5005.

[257] Huang JB, Liu YL, Sun PW, et al.Novel strategy for treatment of pulmonary hypertension: enhancement of apoptosis.*Lung.* 2010;188:179-89.

[258] Emin G, Xiao S. The key role of apoptosis in the pathogenesis and treatment of pulmonary hypertension. *European Journal of Cardio-thoracic Surgery* 2006;30:499—507.

In: Pulmonary Hypertension
Editor: Huili Gan

ISBN: 978-1-61470-556-7
© 2012 Nova Science Publishers, Inc.

Chapter II

Possible Bridging to Final Repair in Eisenmenger Syndrome

Ming-Tai Lin[1] and Yih-Sharng Chen[2]
Department of Pediatrics[1] and Surgery[2], National Taiwan University Hospital, Taipei, Taiwan

Abstract

1. Congenital heart disease (CHD)-related pulmonary arterial hypertension (PAH) remains a major concern despite advances in cardiac surgery. The currently accepted mechanism of CHD-related PAH holds that increased pulmonary blood flow and pressure trigger unfavorable vascular remodeling. Eisenmenger syndrome (ES), the most advanced form, is defined as CHD with an initially large systemic-to-pulmonary shunt, that induces severe pulmonary vascular disease and PAH, with resultant reversal of the shunt and central cyanosis. Eisenmenger syndrome (ES) is usually considered inoperable, but recent success of advanced vasodilator therapies for idiopathic PAH has offered new hope for ES patients.

2. This review initially provides an overview of the pathophysiology of ES and then an evaluation of differences between ES and other forms of PAH, including increased survival, more effective adaptation of RV, polyclonal endothelial cell proliferation, and less occurrence of mutations in the Type II bone morphogenetic protein receptor. Up to one third of ES patients demonstrated maintaining some degree of pulmonary vasoreactivity.

3. With increased understanding of the mechanisms of developing ES, several targeted therapies for PAH associated with CHD, including endothelin receptor antagonists and phosphodiesterase Type-5 inhibitors, have been proved to be effective in reducing pulmonary vascular resistance and symptoms. Pairs of staged surgical approaches aimed to reverse vascular remodeling, such as pulmonary arterial band, one-way flap and Mustard operation, have also been attempted to limit flow and shear stress on pulmonary circulation. Some selected patients exhibited promising improvement in functional class and even achieved final total repair. In this paper, we review the small-scale advanced studies and classify them, in an anatomic manner, into pre-tricuspid, post-tricuspid and complex types of CHD. Size of the defect, magnitude of the shunt, changes of vascular resistance, pulmonary pressure, saturation and exercise tolerance, and percentages of achievement of final repair are summarized and discussed. Further large-scale prospective investigations are required to elucidate both the benefits of these novel approaches in ES and the optimal time for initiating treatment.

Background

In 1897, Dr. Eisenmenger described a 32-year-old man with cyanosis and hemoptysis who was found to have a large ventricular septal defect (VSD) after death [1]. Dr. Wood raised the term "Eisenmenger syndrome" to represent the most advanced from of pulmonary arterial hypertension (PAH) associated with congenital heart defects (CHD) [2]. Currently, Eisenmenger syndrome (ES) is defined as CHD with an initially large systemic-to-pulmonary shunt that induces severe pulmonary vascular disease and PAH, with resultant reversal of the shunt and central cyanosis. Despite recent advances in neonatal cardiac surgery, PAH associated with CHD remains a major concern, even in developed countries. In a recent survey [3], the prevalence of PAH among 1,824 adult CHD patients with septal defect was 6.1 %, whereas 3.5 % of them had ES. Eisenmenger syndrome (ES) is usually considered inoperable and its management has traditionally focused on palliative and supportive treatment. However, combined with increased understanding of pathophysiology of ES, the success of targeted vasodilator therapy in reducing PAH and pulmonary vascular resistance has offered new hope and therapeutic options for patients with ES. This paper provides an overview of the pathophysiology of ES and evaluation of differences between ES and other forms of PAH. We also examine the key data on emerging medical and surgical treatments to reduce pulmonary arterial resistance in patients with ES. For convenience and consistency of discussion, we define severe PAH as the ratio of mean pulmonary arterial pressure to mean blood pressure being more than 0.7, and ES as CHD with systemic pulmonary pressure and cyanosis.

Pathophysiology of Eisenmenger Syndrome (ES)

Eisenmenger syndrome (ES) is the most advanced form of PAH associated with CHD. The histopathologic features of PAH, in such scenarios, include medial hypertrophy with hyperplasia of smooth muscle cells and an increase in connective tissue and elastic fibers, extension of smooth muscles into peripheral pulmonary arteries, intimal and adventitial thickening, and plumbing of the pulmonary arterial tree [4-6]. Complex plexiform lesions, which are a focal proliferation of endothelial channels lined by myofibroblasts, smooth muscles cells, and connective tissue matrices, may also develop. Anatomical changes are progressive, related to PAH severity, and, though reversible at an early stage, can become severe and irreversible when the opportunity for repair is missed.

The pathogenesis of these changes in ES is thought to be multifactorial and similar to those observed in other forms of PAH [4,7,8]. At the early stages of CHD with systemic-to-pulmonary shunts, high blood flow and pressure through the pulmonary circulation result in shear stress and circumferential stress, which exert on the pulmonary endothelium and induce endothelial dysfunction and pulmonary vasoconstriction [9]. Endothelial dysfunction leads to: (1) chronically impaired production of vasodilators, such as nitric oxide and prostacyclin [10]; (2) overexpression of vasoconstrictors, such as thromboxane [11] and endothelin [12]; (3) increased turnover of serotonin; and (4) altered expression of potassium channels [6]. Many of these abnormalities further raise vascular tone and promote vascular remodeling. Such processes involve several cell types in all three layers of pulmonary vessels, including endothelial cells, smooth muscle cells, inflammatory cells, and fibroblasts [5,13]. Moreover, enhanced expression of transforming growth factor-β1 (TGF-β1), platelet derived growth factor (PDGF), and fibroblast growth factor-2 (FGF-2) has been demonstrated in lambs with increased pulmonary blood flow and pulmonary hypertension [14–16]. In addition to being pro-inflammatory, TGF-β1 is an essential profibrotic cytokine [17] that leads to increased production of extracellular matrix, including collagen, elastin, and fibronectin observed in the adventitia of pulmonary arterioles in ES patients.

Interplay of the biomolecules contributes to the characteristic proliferative and obstructive changes of pulmonary vasculature (for example, plexiform lesions) in ES patients.

Structural changes in the pulmonary vasculature are qualitatively similar in various forms of PAH, including ES [5]. Actually, in the Venice classification, PAH associated with CHD is grouped with idiopathic, drug-, connective tissue disease- and human immunodeficiency virus–related etiologies [18]. However, several vascular differences between patients with ES and IPAH have been reported [19]. Differences may exist at tissue, cellular, genetic, and molecular levels between disorders in Category 1 that remain to be elucidated. For instance, Dr. Hall [20] studied lung biopsies from CHD children with pulmonary vascular disease and suggested that, different from idiopathic PAH, their pulmonary circulation does not grow normally. In fact, intra-acinar arteries are reduced, and endothelial dysfunction and smooth muscle cell hyperplasia are present early after birth. Therefore, fundamental differences in pathophysiology are likely to be present in ES and idiopathic patients.

Lee et al. [21] assessed the methylation pattern of the human androgen receptor gene by PCR in proliferated endothelial cells in plexiform lesions from female primary pulmonary hypertension (primary PH) patients (n=4) compared with secondary pulmonary hypertension (secondary PH) patients (n=4). In primary PH, 17 of 22 lesions (77%) were monoclonal. However, in secondary PH, all 19 lesions examined were polyclonal. Smooth muscle cell hyperplasia in pulmonary vessels (n=11) in primary and secondary PH was shown to be polyclonal in all but one of the examined vessels. The monoclonal expansion of endothelial cells provides the first marker that allows the distinction between primary and secondary PH and the monoclonal endothelial cell proliferation detected in PPH suggests that a somatic genetic alteration similar to that present in neoplastic processes may represent the underlying factor that allows a clonal expansion of pulmonary endothelial cells. Such polyclonal findings in CHD patients with PAH also seemed to echo the results of PAH-related genetic studies. For example, mutations in bone morphogenetic protein receptor Type 2 are less common in patients with pulmonary hypertensive congenital heart disease than idiopathic pulmonary hypertension, but when present might profoundly influence outcome [22-24]. These differences may result from the initial preservation of right ventricular function and relief of excess pressure via the right-to-left shunt [24].

A previous study reported extensive evaluations of ventricular morphology in patients with ES, a group with left-to-right shunt VSD and mild elevation of pulmonary arterial pressure, and fetuses with healthy hearts [24,25]. They found the same ventricular morphology in all three groups—a flat ventricular septum and equal thickness of the right and left ventricular free walls. They, therefore, suggested that the usual regression of RV wall thickness after birth does not occur in the presence of large shunts; and RV retains function even with increased mechanical demand.

Evaluation of Operability

Consideration of closure of a defect with the left-to-right shunt involves the amount of cardiac output, the size and location of the defect, the degree of shunt, and vasoreactivity of pulmonary circulation. Herein, we summarize the available tools and parameters as follows.

1. Hemodynamic assessment by cardiac catheterization :
   Pulmonary vascular resistance (PVR) > 10 woods unit. m^2 is thought to be relatively poor in candidates for defect closure because of high risk of sustained pulmonary hypertension, right heart failure, and pulmonary hypertension crisis [26]. A suggested pulmonary-to-systemic ratio of resistance (Rp/Rs <0.7) and/or further decline of this index to 0.42 were favorable for operation [26,27].
2. Pulmonary vaso-reactivity :
   Inhaled 100 % oxygen, via a rebreathing mask, was the most commonly used agent [26]. During recent years, acute vasodilator testing with short-acting vasodilators, such as inhaled nitric oxide (NO), intravenous epoprostenol, and adenosine, have been used. Positive response was defined as a 20 % decrease of pulmonary pressure.
3. Lung biopsy :
   Drs. Heath and Edward [4] published their observations and described six grades of pulmonary vascular disease in 1958. They further correlated such a grading system and results to hemodynamic findings [8] and immediate reversibility [28] of pulmonary hypertension in patients with cardiac septal defect. To further distinguish patients not suitable for defect closure, several scoring systems were proposed. Rabinovitch

[29,30] and Haworth [31,32] have adopted morphometric approaches and added some modification to the classification by Drs. Heath and Edward. A Japanese group designed the so-called index of pulmonary vascular disease (IPVD) and suggested an IPVD rating of 2.1 as upper permissible limits for defect closure [33,34]. This grading system provides qualitative information about plexogenic pulmonary arteriopathy and receives widespread clinical use.

4. Test occlusion :

During the procedure of percutaneous transcatheter closure of the left-to-right shunt, balloon test occlusion may signal reversibility of PAH and provide additional information on the suitability for closure and the possible post-procedural outcome [35].

Attempts to Increase Operability of ES Patients

With increased understanding of mechanisms for developing ES, several targeted therapies for PAH associated with CHD have proved effective in reducing pulmonary vascular resistance and symptoms. Pairs of staged surgical approaches aimed to reverse vascular remodeling were also attempted to limit flow and shear stress on pulmonary circulation. Some selected patients exhibited promising improvement in functional class and even achieved final total repair. In this section, we review small-scale advanced studies and classify them, in an anatomic manner, into pre-tricuspid, post-tricuspid, and complex types of CHD.

Medical Attempt

In the past 15 years [9,36], multiple randomized controlled studies have demonstrated the efficacy of three classes of drugs for the treatment of PAH patients, namely: (i) prostanoids; (ii) endothelin receptor antagonists; and (iii) phosphodiesterase (PDE)-5 inhibitors. The rationale supporting the use of these drugs in CHD patients with pulmonary hypertension is based on the similarities between pulmonary vascular changes observed in ES and in other forms of PAH. Unfortunately, only a few randomized controlled studies have included patients with PAH associated with repaired or unrepaired CHD [37-40], and the sub-group analysis appears less reliable for such a small number of patients. There were also several small-scale studies of the three groups of targeted therapies, alone or in combinations, which have shown improvements in exercise capacity, functional class and even hemodynamic data without safety issues [36,41-43]. Here, we do not plan to describe these studies one-by-one. We describe two randomized, double-blind, placebo-controlled study focused on patients with ES: the BREATHE-5 (Bosentan Randomized Trial of Endothelin Antagonist Therapy-5) study [44] and EARLY study [45]. At baseline, all patients in the BREATHE-5 study, including children (patients > 12 years), were in functional class III. The study showed a statistically significant treatment effect for reduction of the pulmonary vascular resistance index and decrease of the mean pulmonary arterial pressure. Remarkable in this trial was the increased pulmonary vascular resistance index observed in the placebo arm. This elevation in functional class III patients in a small period of time, 16 weeks, was not expected. The 6MWD resulted in a treatment effect of 53 m (P = 0.008). Directly after the end of this study, a subgroup was included in an extension prospective cohort study. This 6MWD data showed improvement in those patients who had initially received placebo (33 m) and maintenance of the effect in patients who were treated with bosentan (67 m) [44]. Bosentan was well tolerated and did not adversely affect systemic arterial oxygen saturation. Safety and tolerability of long-term use of Bosentan are still under investigation.

Another randomized controlled trial investigating bosentan was the EARLY study by Galiè et al [45] about bosentan treatment exclusively on PAH patients in functional class II. A subgroup of CHD-PAH patients (n = 32) were analyzed. Increase in 6MWD was demonstrated at 6 months from baseline, but the changes were not statistically significant. Bosentan treatment was associated with a lower incidence of decline in functional class compared to placebo (P = 0.03).

Surgical Attempt

Aside from palliative procedures, current practice provides another three surgical options for such ES patients: lung transplantation with intracardiac repair, heart-lung transplantation, and high-risk intracardiac repair. However, mortality and morbidity are not presently low. Therefore, various types of surgical efforts were attempted to change the natural course of CHD patients with PAH.

Generally, if the congenital heart defect is repaired before the age of 2, abnormal pulmonary vascular remodeling is generally reversible [29]. However, not all lesions have the same propensity to cause pulmonary vascular disease [46]. For example, individuals with large VSDs and patent ductus arteriosus are more likely to develop severe PAH at a faster rate, compared to ASDs; in which, if PAH develops, it does so later in life [47]. Additionally, patients with TGA and VSD or truncus arteriosus develop severe pulmonary vascular disease even earlier, usually during the first year of life. By contrast, pulmonary pressure in patients with an isolated large VSD or PDA increases gradually over time, but rarely reaches the systemic level before the age of 2.

#ASD

In pre-tricuspid shunts such as ASD, initial systemic-to-pulmonary shunting induces an increase in pulmonary blood flow and a mild elevation in pulmonary arterial pressure with normal or reduced PVR (hyperkinetic pulmonary circulation). Based on the 5-year follow-up data from the Euro Heart Survey [48] on adult congenital heart disease (ACHD), 1,877 patients were enrolled for analysis, 896 of them exhibited an ASD, and 710 of them exhibited VSD. Prevalence of ES in the adult ASD patients was significantly lower than that in the adult VSD patients (15/896 and 83/710, $p<0.001$).

Although the possibility of developing severe pulmonary hypertension or ES is relatively lower, closure of ASD is still necessary for such ASD patients because, without treatment, the incidence of atrial arrhythmia, stroke, and sudden death increases. Furthermore, unfavorable postoperative courses occur in some elderly ASD patients [49]. Data regarding closure of ASD in the presence of severe pulmonary hypertension are relatively scarce and limited to small series reports. We classify these reports according to the palliative strategy used: (1) shunt closure with preceding targeted therapies; and (2) fenestrated ASD occluder.

(1) Shunt Closure with Preceding Targeted Therapies

Imanaka et al. [50] reported a 51-year-old patient with ASD and severe PAH. Despite high pulmonary pressure and vascular resistance, he underwent ASD closure because OP/QS of 2.0 was demonstrated. Nitric oxide was administered to treat severe postoperative pulmonary hypertension crisis. Finally, the patient improved, having eventually received clinical and hemodynamic treatment. Since 1998, several groups have reported experiences of defect closure with preceding use of prostaglandin I_2 [51–53] or Sidenafil [54], and have demonstrated improvement of functional class and decline of pulmonary pressure [Table 1].

Table 1. Results of ASD closure and targeted therapies in adult patients

	Year published	Age (years)	Baseline MPAP (mm Hg)	Medication Type	Duration (months)	Improvement(Y/N) Clinical	Hemo dynamic
Schwerzmann et al.	2006	38	53	PGI_2	12	Y	Y
Yamauchi et al.	2001	35	65	PGI_2	24	Y	Y
Frost et al.	2005	29	60	PGI_2	48	Y	Y
Imanaka et al.	1998	51	53	NO	–	Y	Y
Kim et al.	2010	41	?	Sidenatil	48	Y	Y

MPAP: Mean pulmonary artery pressure; NYHA: New York Heart Association; ASD: article septal defect; PDA: patent ductus arteriosus; NO: nitric oxide; PGI_2: prostacyclin.

(2) Fenestrated ASD Occluder

Considering different ASD-related RV/LV physiology, especially at advanced age, such modified and incomplete ASD occlusion was proposed to allow "decompression" for an overflow of blood in both directions if ventricular diastolic or systolic dysfunction is present. The use of fenestrated ASD devices was first evaluated in animal studies in 2002 [55]. Thereafter, Holzer et al. [56], described their first experience of ASD closure with self-fabricated fenestrated Amplatzer septal occluder in an 86-year-old patient. During the procedure, test occlusion resulted in significant elevation of left atrial pressure (12→32mmHg) and the procedure was, therefore, abandoned. Two months later, the patient was re-admitted and underwent ASD closure with a self-fabricated fenestrated device (size of fenestration: 6 mm). Post-catheterization course was uneventful . In 2007, Bruch et al. [57] described an experience of deploying fenestrated Amplatzer septal occluders in 15 ASD patients (48–77 years old) with significant pulmonary hypertension (mean PAP: 25–50mmHg). Catheterization 1year after closure showed decreased (12/15) or similar (3/15) pulmonary artery pressure. Functional class of all 15 patients improved. These limited promising short-term results might suggest that the fenestrated ASD closure device is an alternative for some high-risk ASD patients, especially those with pulmonary hypertension and/or decreased left ventricular compliance.

#VSD

Post-tricuspid valve left-to-right shunt (similar to VSD) is considered a corrective disease if surgery is performed in the early stages. When severe pulmonary hypertension later develops, especially over ten years, patients are usually considered as a high-risk and unfavorable group to receive direct closure of the shunt [58–60]. However, several studies at the beginning of the 21th century have shown that the unloading of pulmonary hypertension can result in remodeling of the pulmonary vasculature and possible improvement of pulmonary hypertension [61,62]. Research has also shown that pulmonary vascular resistance in some patients with primary or secondary PAH may show significant decrease after long-term vasodilator therapy, even when patients fail to respond to acute dilator tests [63-65]. Therefore, palliative surgery to reduce pulmonary flow, such as pop-off flap, fenestrated patch and pulmonary artery banding (PAB), has also been attempted during the past several decades [66–70].

a. Pop-off Flap and Fenestrated Patch

Novick et al., in 2005 [66], reported an experience of flap valve in 54 children with simple VSD and pulmonary hypertension. Median age and pulmonary vascular resistance of the 54 children were 5.1 year sold (range: 5 months to 17 years) and 11.7(±5.4) Wood units. Percentages of hospital and late death were 2/54 and 2/48 respectively. Later, Zhang et al. [67] also described similar results regarding application of unidirectional monovalve to 27 patients (age: 15.0±5.6 years) with large VSD and PAH (15.2±3.8 Wood units).

b. Pulmonary Artery Banding (PAB)

The use of pulmonary artery banding (PAB) in CHD patients with severe pulmonary hypertension is not new [68–70]. The possible explanation for PAB effectively lowering pulmonary pressure might be: (1) severe pulmonary hypertension in some CHD patients may be related to large flow and long duration of the shunt. The palliative procedure for decreasing the flow to pulmonary vasculature may have a chance of reversing the disease process over a certain period. (2) Pulmonary artery banding (PAB) resulted in a right-to-left shunt with a consequent decrease in the saturation of pulmonary arteries. This may have caused dilatation of the pulmonary vascular bed and a decrease in PVR. Dammann et al. [68] studied a series of 63 VSD patients in 1961, ten of whom were older than 2 years old and had systemic-level pulmonary pressure. Two patients died after PAB from pulmonary hypertension crisis. Another two patients had subsequent intracardiac repair and one of them died perioperatively. Table 2 summarizes several case reports about PAB on older children with VSD and PAH [68–70].

In 2010, we reported [71] our experience of using PAB on young adult patients with VSD and severe pulmonary hypertension. Five such patients (17–34 years) had ratios of mean PAP/mean BP ranged from 0.59 to 1.06. Results of PAB on these patients seemed promising and mean pulmonary pressure decreased significantly (77.5±9.2 mmHg to 42.0±9.0 mmHg). This observation extended the application of PAB in the young adult patients who may have more advanced pulmonary hypertension (even Eisenmenger syndrome) associated with CHD.

Together, these reports seemed to provide an alternative treatment modality for some selected CHD with PAH. Whether all CHD patients with severe pulmonary hypertension should undergo palliative procedure still requires more observations and follow-up.

#TGA/VSD

Currently, arterial switch for d-TGA and Taussig-Bing anomaly has become the preferred surgical procedure and has shown extremely low (2–5 %) early mortality [72,73]. However, some of these children require medical care beyond 6 months of age, when severe pulmonary hypertension might have already established [74]. Rapid elevation of pulmonary pressure might be due to high pulmonary flow, high pulmonary artery pressure, hypoxia or polycythemia [75]. Severe palliative surgical attempts have been performed since 1972, including atrial switch [76–78] and arterial switch [79–82].

Table 2. Result of PAB in patients (>2 years old) with VSD and PAH

Year published	Case number	Age (years)	MPAP* (mm Hg)	MPAP/MBP*	change of SpO2	Hospital death	Post-PAB MPAP/MBP	Reference
1984	2	N/A	N/A	N/A		0	N/A?	69
1997	1	19	70	$^{70}/_{96}$	97%→75%	0	0.5	70
2006	4	3.6.7.13	62.64.75.80	$^{62}/_{70}.$ $^{80}/_{80}$ $^{64}/_{71}./$ $^{75}/_{87}$		0	$^{50}/_{56}.$ $^{18}/_{51}.$ $^{35}/_{56}.$ $^{39}/_{68}$	67

a. Palliative Atrial Switch

Lindesmith et al. [76] first reported application of the Mustard procedure to TGA/VSD patients with late PAH. In addition to 15 % early mortality, symptomatic arrhythmia and baffle obstruction were also noted in the long-term follow-up [83].

Burkhart et al. [77], in 2004, described another series of 28 patients with TGA/VSD or hemodynamically similar complex CHD who underwent palliative atrial switch with the VSDs left open at a median age of 10 years old (range: 1–27). Early mortality rate was 8.7 %, and 5-, 10-, and 15-year survival rates were 84 %, 64 %, and 54%, respectively. Mean postoperative systemic arterial oxygen saturation increased significantly to 88 % from preoperative saturation of 65 %. The New York Heart Association (NYHA) functional class also significantly improved from III~IV to I~II.

b. Arterial Switch

Arterial switch operation (ASO) has become the most effective treatment for infants with TGA and VSD [84,85]. Similar to atrical switch, palliative ASO was also conducted in several older children, previously thought inoperable, to improve systems of such patients. Pridjian et al. [79] and Elizari et al. [80] independently reported experiences of palliative ASO in $5^{1}/_{2}$- and 7-year-old patients. Both reports have described postoperative improvement in saturation and exercise intolerance in these two children. Recently, Lei at al. [81] evaluated the midterm outcomes of palliative ASO in 21 patients with TGA, VSD, and severe PVOD. Mean age and follow-up of enrolled patients were 3.7 years old (range: 0.5–15) and 4 years (range: 0.25–9.5 years). Early mortality was 14.3 % (3/21) and another patient suffered from sudden death 3 months after surgery. Mean systemic arterial oxygen saturation increased significantly from 69 % (preoperative) to 93 % (postoperative). Mean preoperative value of systolic pulmonary arterial pressure was 91 mmHg. Regression of pulmonary pressure occurred in eight of them (8/21:38 %) and three of these eight VSDs were closed later. Functional class of these survival cases improved from III~IV to I~II. This study extended the previous experience of palliative ASO in TGA/VSD patients and first demonstrated the possibility of reversal of pulmonary vascular remodeling. Almost simultaneously, another group [82] from China reported a similarly promising experience regarding 86 patients with TGA/VSD hemodynamics (mean age: 2 years old, range: 0.5–19), 11 of whom exhibited extremely high pulmonary resistance (>8 units. m^2).

The overall (2000–2008) early mortality was 7.0 % (6/86) and decreased surprisingly to zero (0/46) between 2006 and 2008, when "diagnostic-treatment-and-repair" strategy [26] was adopted with advanced use of nitric oxide, sildenafil, and bosentan. Using the targeted therapy, this study further improved the midterm outcome of palliative ASO for patients older than 6 months with TGA/VSD or Taussig-Bing anomaly and severe PAH. Together, the results of the aforementioned studies have indicated that palliative surgery seemed to be practical for such groups of patients. However, long-term benefits, patient selection, and synergistic effect on targeted vasodilator therapy showed be evaluated in large cohort.

Conclusion

Eisenmenger syndrome is usually thought to be synonymous with "inoperable". However, with the progress of advanced medication and surgical attempts, some patients of this group have seemed "inoperable" more no longer. In the future, surgical and other therapeutic approaches aimed at reversing vascular remodeling and regenerating the pulmonary microvasculature may be of benefit to our understanding of ES and the optimal management of ES. Further investigation is required to elucidate the benefits of these novel approaches in ES, the optimal time for initiating intervention, and optimal combinations of various palliative modalities.

Reference

[1] Eisenmenger V. (1897) Die angeborenen Defect der Kammer ssheidew and des Herzens. *Z Klin Med.* 32(suppl 1):1-28.
[2] Wood P. (1958) The Eisenmenger Syndrome: II. *Br Med J.* 2:755-62.
[3] Duffels MGJ, Engelfriet PM, Berger RMF, et al. (2007) Pulmonary arterial hypertension in congenital heart disease: an epidemiologic perspective from a Dutch registry. *Int J Cardiol.* 120:198-204.
[4] Heath D, Edwards JE. (1958) The pathology of hypertensive pulmonary vascular disease: a description of six grades of structural changes in the pulmonary arteries with special reference to congenital cardiac septal defects. *Circulation.* 18:533–47.
[5] Pietra GG, Capron F, Stewart S, et al. (2004) Pathologic assessment of vasculopathies in pulmonary hypertension. *J Am Coll Cardiol.* 43 Suppl S:25S–32S.
[6] Diller GP, Gatzoulis MA. (2007) Pulmonary vascular disease in adults with congenital heart disease. *Circulation.* 115:1039–50.
[7] Dimopoulos K, Giannakoulas G, Wort SJ, Gatzoulis MA. (2008) Pulmonary arterial hypertension in adults with congenital heart disease: distinct differences from other causes of pulmonary arterial hypertension and management implications. *Curr Opin Cardiol.* Nov;23(6):545-54.
[8] Heath D, Helmholz HFJ, Burchell HB, Dushane JW, Edwards JE. (1958) Graded pulmonary vascular changes and hemodynamic findings in cases of atrial and ventricular septal defect and patent ductus arteriosus. *Circulation.* 18:1155–66.
[9] Beghetti M, Galiè N. (2009) Eisenmenger syndrome a clinical perspective in a new therapeutic era of pulmonary arterial hypertension. *J Am Coll Cardiol.* Mar 3;53(9):733-40. Review.
[10] Budhiraja R, Tuder RM, Hassoun PM. (2004) Endothelial dysfunction in pulmonary hypertension. *Circulation.* 109:159-65.
[11] Adatia I, Barrow SE, Stratton PD, Ritter JM, Haworth SG. (1994) Effect of intracardiac repair on biosynthesis of thromboxane A2 and prostacyclin in children with a left to right shunt. *Br Heart J.* 72:452-456.
[12] Stewart DJ, Levy RD, Cernacek P, Langleben D. (1991) Increased plasma endothelin-1 in pulmonary hypertension: marker or mediator of disease? *Ann Intern Med.* 114:464-469.

[13] Humbert M, Morrell N, Archer S, et al. (2004) Cellular and molecular pathobiology of pulmonary arterial hypertension. *J Am Coll Cardiol.* 43:S13-24.
[14] Mata-Greenwood E, Meyrick B, Steinhorn RH, Fineman JR, Black SM. (2003) Alterations in TGF-beta1 expression in lambs with increased pulmonary blood flow and pulmonary hypertension. *Am J Physiol Lung Cell Mol Physiol.* 285:L209-L221.
[15] Mata-Greenwood E , Meyrick B , Soifer SJ , Fineman JR , Black SM. (2003) Expression of VEGF and its receptors Flt-1 and Flk-1/KDR is altered in lambs with increased pulmonary blood fl ow and pulmonary hypertension. *Am J Physiol Lung Cell Mol Physiol.* 285:L222-L231.
[16] Wedgwood S , Devol JM , Grobe A , et al. (2007) Fibroblast growth factor-2 expression is altered in lambs with increased pulmonary blood flow and pulmonary hypertension. *Pediatr Res.* 61:32-36.
[17] Wynn TA. (2007) Common and unique mechanisms regulate fibrosis in various fibroproliferative diseases. *JCI.* 117:524-9.
[18] Simonneau G, Galiè N, Rubin LJ, et al. (2004) Clinical classification of pulmonary hypertension. *J Am Coll Cardiol.* 43(Suppl):5S-12S.
[19] Sheehan R, Perloff JK, Fishbein MC, Gjertson D, Aberle DR. (2005) Pulmonary neovascularity: a distinctive radiographic finding in Eisenmenger syndrome. *Circulation.* 112:2778–85.
[20] Hall SM, Haworth SG. (1992) Onset and evolution of pulmonary vascular disease in young children: abnormal postnatal remodelling studied in lung biopsies. *J Pathol.* 166:183–93.
[21] Lee S-D, Shroyer KR, Markham NE, Cool CD, Voelkel NF, Tuder RM. (1998) Monoclonal endothelial cell proliferation is present in primary but not secondary pulmonary hypertension. *J Clin Invest.* 101:927-934.
[22] Roberts KE, McElroy JJ, Wong WP, et al. (2004) BMPR2 mutations in pulmonary arterial hypertension with congenital heart disease. *Eur Respir J.* 24:371- 374.
[23] Harrison RE, Berger R, Haworth SG, et al. (2005) Transforming growth factor-beta receptor mutations and pulmonary arterial hypertension in childhood. *Circulation.* 111:435-441.
[24] Hopkins WE, Waggoner AD. (2002) Severe pulmonary hypertension without right ventricular failure: the unique hearts of patients with Eisenmenger syndrome. *Am J Cardiol.* 89:34-8.

[25] Hopkins WE, Ochoa LL, Richardson GW, Trulock EP. (1996) Comparison of the hemodynamics and survival of adults with severe primary pulmonary hypertension or Eisenmenger syndrome. *J Heart Lung Transplant.* 15:100-5.

[26] Dimopoulos K, Peset A, Gatzolius MA. (2008) Evaluating operability in adults with congenital heart disease and the role of pretreatment with targeted pulmonary arterial hypertension therapy. (2008) *Int J Cardiol.* 129:163-71.

[27] Balzer DT, Kort HW, Day RW, et al. (2002) Inhaled nitric oxide as a preoperative test (INOP Test I): the INOP Test Study Group. *Circulation.* 106(Suppl):I76–81.

[28] Heath D, Helmholz HFJ, Burchell HB, Dushane JW, Kirklin JW, Edwards JE. (1958) Relation between structural changes in the small pulmonary arteries and the immediate reversibility of pulmonary hypertension following closure of ventricular and atrial septal defects. *Circulation.* 18:1167–74.

[29] Rabinovitch M, Haworth SG, Castaneda AR, Nadas AS, Reid LM. (1978) Lung biopsy in congenital heart disease: a morphometric approach to pulmonary vascular disease. *Circulation.* 58(6):1107–1122.

[30] Rabinovitch M, Keane JF, Norwood WI, Castaneda AR, Reid L. (1984) Vascular structure in lung tissue obtained at biopsy correlated with pulmonary hemodynamic findings after repair of congenital heart defects. *Circulation.* 69(4):655–667.

[31] Haworth SG. (1987) Pulmonary vascular disease in ventricular septal defect: structural and functional correlations in lung biopsies from 85 patients, with outcome of intracardiac repair. *J Pathol.* 152(3):157–168.

[32] Haworth SG, Hislop AA. (1983) Pulmonary vascular development: normal values of peripheral vascular structure. *Am J Cardiol.* 52:578-583.

[33] Yamaki S, Mohri H, Haneda K, Endo M, Akimoto H. (1989) Indications for surgery based on lung biopsy in cases of ventricular septal defect and/or patent ductus arteriosus with severe pulmonary hypertension. *Chest.* 96:31-39.

[34] Yamakis, Tezuka F. (1976) Quantitative Analysis of Pulmonary Vascular Disease in Complete Transposition of the Great Arteries. *Circulation.* 54:805-9.

[35] Jaiyesimi F, Ruberu DK, Misra VK.(1993) Pattern of congenital heart disease in Kingfahd specialist hospital, Buraidah. *Ann Saudi Med.* 13:407-11.

[36] Schuuring MJ, Vis JC, Duffels MG, Bouma BJ, Mulder BJ. (2010) Adult patients with pulmonary arterial hypertension due to congenital heart disease: a review on advanced medical treatment with bosentan. *Ther Clin Risk Manag.* 6:359-66.

[37] Simonneau G, Barst RJ, Galie N, et al. (2002) Continuous subcutaneous infusion of treprostinil, a prostacyclin analogue, in patients with pulmonary arterial hypertension. a double-blind, randomized, placebo-controlled trial. *Am J Respir Crit Care Med.* 165: 800-4.
[38] Rubin LJ, Badesch DB, Barst RJ, et al. (2002) Bosentan therapy for pulmonary arterial hypertension. *N Engl J Med.* 346:896-903.
[39] Galie N, Humbert M, Vachiery JL, et al. (2002) Effects of beraprost sodium, an oral prostacyclin analogue, in patients with pulmonary arterial hypertension: a randomised, double-blind placebo-controlled trial. *J Am Coll Cardiol.* 39: 1496-502.
[40] Barst RJ, Langleben D, Badesch D, et al. (2006) Treatment of pulmonary arterial hypertension with the selective endothelin-a receptor antagonist sitaxsentan. *J Am Coll Cardiol.* 47:2049-56.
[41] Mukhopadhyay S, Sharma M, Ramakrishnan S, et al. (2006) Phosphodiesterase-5 inhibitor in Eisenmenger syndrome: a preliminary observational study. *Circulation.* 114:1807–10.
[42] Lu XL, Xiong CM, Shan GL, et al. (2010) Impact of sildenafil therapy on pulmonary arterial hypertension in adults with congenital heart disease. *Cardiovasc Ther.* 2010 Dec;28(6):350-5.
[43] D'Alto M, Romeo E, Argiento P, et al. (2010) Bosentan-sildenafil association in patients with congenital heart disease-related pulmonary arterial hypertension and Eisenmenger physiology. *Int J Cardiol.* Nov 15. [Epub ahead of print]
[44] Galiè N, Beghetti M, Gatzoulis MA, et al. (2006) Bosentan therapy in patients with Eisenmenger syndrome: a multicenter, double-blind, randomized, lacebo-controlled study. *Circulation.* 114:48 –54.
[45] 45.Galie N, Rubin LJ, Hoeper MM et al. (2008) Treatment of patients with mildly symptomatic pulmonary arterial hypertension with bosentan (EARLY study): a double-blind, randomised controlled trial. *The Lancet.* 371:2093-2100.
[46] Beghetti M. (2006) *Pulmonary arterial hypertension related to congenital heart disease.* Munich: Elsevier.
[47] Vogel M, Berger F, Kramer A, Alexi-Meshkishvili V, Lange PE. (1999) Incidence of secondary pulmonary hypertension in adults with atrial septal or sinus venosus defects. *Heart.* 82:30-33.
[48] Engelfriet PM, Duffels MG, Möller T, et al. (2007) Pulmonary arterial hypertension in adults born with a heart septal defect: the Euro Heart Survey on adult congenital heart disease. *Heart.* 93:682-7.

[49] Ghosh S, Chatterjee S, Black E, et al. (2002) Surgical closure of atrial septal defects in adults: effect of age at operation on outcome. *Heart.* 88:485–7.
[50] Imanaka K, Kotsuka Y, Takamoto S, Furuse A, Inoue K, Shirai T. (1998) Atrial septal defect and severe pulmonary hypertension in an adult who needed nitric oxide inhalation after repair. *Kyobu Geka.* 51:403–5.
[51] Schwerzmann M, Zafar M, McLaughlin PR, Chamberlain DW, Webb G, Granton J. (2006) Atrial septal defect closure in a patient with "irreversible" pulmonary hypertensive arteriopathy. *Int J Cardiol.* 110:104–7.
[52] Gatzoulis MA, Beghetti M, Galie N, et al. (2008) Longer-term bosentan therapy improves functional capacity in Eisenmenger syndrome: results of the BREATHE-5 open-label extension study. *Int J Cardiol.* 127:27-32.
[53] Yamauchi H, Yamaki S, Fujii M, Iwaki H, Tanaka S. (2001) Reduction in recalcitrant pulmonary hypertension after operation for atrial septal defect. *Ann Thorac Surg.* 72:905–6.
[54] Kim YH, Yu JJ, Yun TJ, et al. (2010) Repair of Atrial Septal Defect With Eisenmenger Syndrome After Long-Term Sildenafil Therapy. *Ann Thorac Surg.* 89:1629–30.
[55] Kong H, Gu X, Titus JL, et al. (2002) Creation of an intra-atrial communication with a new Amplatzer shunt prosthesis: Preliminary results in a swine model. *Catheter Cardiovasc Interv.* 56:267-271.
[56] Holzer R, Cao QL, Hijazi ZM. (2005) Closure of a moderately large atrial septal defect with a self-fabricated fenestrated amplatzer septal occlude in an 85-year-old patient with reduced diastolic elasticity of the left ventricle. *Catheter Cardiovasc Interv.* 64:513-8.
[57] Bruch L, Winkelmann A, Sonntag S, et al. (2008) Fenestrated occluders for treatment of ASD in elserly patients with pulmonary hypertension and/or right heart failure. *J of Interv Cardiol.* 21(1):44-49.
[58] Friedli B, Kidd BS, Mustard WT, Keith JD. (1974) Ventricular septal defect with increased pulmonary vascular resistance. Late results of surgical closure. *Am J Cardiol.* 33:403–9.
[59] John S, Korula R, Jairaj PS, et al. (1983) Results of surgical treatment of ventricular septal defects with pulmonary hypertension. *Thorax.* 38:279–83.
[60] Bando K, Turrentine MW, Sun K, et al. (1995) Surgical management of complete atrioventricular septal defects. A twenty-year experience. *J Thorac Cardiovasc Surg.* 110:1543–52

[61] O'Blenes SB, Fischer S, McIntyre B, Keshavjee S, Rabinovitch M. (2001) Hemodynamic unloading leads to regression of pulmonary vascular disease in rats. *J Thorac Cardiovasc Surg.* 121:279–289.
[62] Cowan KN, Jones PL, Rabinovitch M. (1999) Regression of hypertrophied rat pulmonary arteries in organ culture is associated with suppression of proteolytic activity, inhibition of tenascin-C, and smooth muscle cell apoptosis. *Circ Res.* 84:1223–1233.
[63] Rosenzweig EB, Kerstein D, Barst RJ. (1999) Long-term prostacyclin for pulmonary hypertension with associated congenital heart defects. *Circulation.* 99:1858–1865.
[64] McLaughlin VV, Genthner DE, Panella MM, Hess DM, Rich S. (1999) Compassionate use of continuous prostacyclin in the management of secondary pulmonary hypertension: a case series. *Ann Intern Med.* 130:740–743.
[65] Barst RJ, Rubin LJ, Long WA, et al. (1996) A comparison of continuous intravenous epoprostenol (prostacyclin) with conventional therapy for primary pulmonary hypertension. *N Engl J Med.* 334:296–301.
[66] Novick WM, Sandoval N, Lazorhysynets VV, et al. (2005) Flap valve double patch closure of ventricular septal defects in children with increased pulmonary vascular resistance. *Ann Thorac Surg.* 79:21–8.
[67] Zhang B, Wu S, Liang J, et al. (2007) Unidirectional monovalve homologous aortic patch for repair of ventricular septal defect with pulmonary hypertension. *Ann Thorac Surg.* 83:2176–81.
[68] Dammann JF, McEachen JA, Thompson WM, Smith R, Muller WH. (1961) The regression of pulmonary vascular disease after creation of pulmonary stenosis. *J Thorac Cardiovasc Surg.* 42:722–734.
[69] Wagenvoort CA, Wagenvoort N. (1984) Reversibility of plexogenic pulmonary arteriopathy following banding of the pulmonary artery. *J Thorac Cardiovasc Surg.* 87:876–886.
[70] Batista RJ, Santos JL, Takeshita N, et al. (1997) Successful reversal of pulmonary hypertension in Eisenmenger complex. *Arq Bras Cardiol.* 68:279–80.
[71] Lin MT, Chen YS, Huang SC, et al. (2010) Alternative approach for selected severe pulmonary hypertension of congenital heart defect without initial correction - Palliative surgical treatment. *Int J Cardiol.* Jun 24. [Epub ahead of print]

[72] Kirklin JW, Blackstone EH, Tchervenkov CI, Castaneda AR, the Congenital Heart Surgeons Society. (1992) Clinical Outcomes After the Arterial Switch Operation for Transposition: Patient, Support, Procedural, and Institutional Risk Factors. *Circulation.* 86:1501-15.
[73] Wernovsky G, Mayer JE, Jonas RA, Hanley FL, Blackstone EH, Kirklin JW, et al. Factors influencing early and late outcome of arterial switch operation for transposition of the great arteries. (1995) *J Thorac Cardiovasc Surg.* 109:289-302.
[74] Hoffman JI, Rudolph AM, Heymann MA. (1981) Pulmonary vascular disease with congenital heart lesions: pathologic features and causes. *Circulation.* 64:873-7.
[75] Clarkson PM, Neutze JM, Wardill JC, Barratt-boyes BG. (1976) The Pulmonary Vascular Bed in Patients with Complete Transposition of the Great Arteries. *Circulation.* 53:539-43.
[76] Lindesmith GG, Stiles QR, Tucker BL, Gallaher ME, Stanton RE, Meyer BW. (1972) The Mustard operation as a palliative procedure. *J Thorac Cardiovasc Surg.* 63:75-80.
[77] Burkhart HM, Dearani JA, Williams WG, et al. (2004) Late result of palliative atrial switch for transposition, ventricular septal defect, and pulmonary vascular obstructive disease. *Ann Thorac Surg.* 77:464-9.
[78] Nakajima Y, Momma K, Seguchi M, Nakazawa M, Imai Y. (1996) Polmonary hypertension in patients with complex transposition of the great arteries: midterm results after surgery. *Pediatr Cardiol.* 17:104-7.
[79] Pridjian AK, Tacy TA, Teske D, Bove EL. (1992) Palliative arterial repair for transposition, ventricular septal defect, and pulmonary vascular obstructive disease. *Ann Thorac Surg.* 54:355-6.
[80] Elizari A, Somerville J. (1999) Palliative arterial switch for complex transposition with ventricular septal defect. *Cardiol Young.* 3:315-8.
[81] Lei BF, Chen JM, Cen JZ, Lui RC, Ding YQ, Xu G, et al. (2010) Palliative arterial switch for transposition of the great arteries, ventricular septal defect, and pulmonary vascular obstructive disease: midterm outcomes. *J Thorac Cardiovasc Surg.* 140:845-9.
[82] Liu YL, Hu SS, Shen XD, et al. (2010) Midterm results of arterial switch operation in older patients with severe pulmonary hypertension. *Ann Thorac Surg.* 90:848-55.
[83] Sagin-Saylam G, Somerville J. (1996) Palliative Mustard operation for transposition of the great arteries: late results after 15-20 years. *Heart.* 75:72-7.

[84] Bical O, hazan E, Lecompte Y, et al. (1984) Anatomic correction of transposition of the great arteries associated with ventricular septal defect. Midterm result in 50 patients. *Circulation.* 70:891-7.

[85] Serraf A, Bruniaux J, Lacour-Gayet F, et al. (1991) Aatomic correction of transposition of the great arteries associated with ventricular septal defect: experience with 117 cases. *J Thorac Cardiovasc Surg.* 102:140-7.

In: Pulmonary Hypertension
Editor: Huili Gan
ISBN: 978-1-61470-556-7
© 2012 Nova Science Publishers, Inc.

Chapter III

The Management of Congenital Systemic-to-Pulmonary Shunt and Advanced Pulmonary Artery Hypertension

Hui-Li Gan[*] *and Jian-Qun Zhang*

Department of Cardiac Surgery, Beijing Anzhen Hospital, Capital Medical University, Beijing Institute of Heart, Lung and Blood Vessel Diseases, Beijing, China

Abstract

Background

Our objective was to investigate the relationship between the long-term survival of surgical treatment and preoperative pulmonary vascular resistance (PVR) and pulmonary to systemic flow ratio (Qp/Qs) in congenital systemic-to-pulmonary shunt with andadvanced pulmonary hypertension.

---

[*] Corresponding Author: Hui-Li Gan, MD, PhD, Cardiac Surgery Department, Beijing Anzhen Hospital, Capital Medical University, Beijing Institute of Heart, Lung and Blood Vessel Diseases, Beijing 100029 China (Tel: +86-10-64456885; Fax: +86-10-62244207 Email: ganhuili@hotmail.com).

Methods and results

1212 cases of congenital systemic-to-pulmonary shunt and advanced pulmonary hypertension were treated non-surgically or surgically and were entered into non-surgical group (n=297) and surgical group (n=915).Propensity score of inclusion into surgical group were estimated and 245 pairs were get with the propensity score matching between the two groups. Results: In the 245 propensity score matched pairs, the actuarial survival at 10 and 15 yrs of the surgical group was significantly higher than that of the non-surgical group when PVR was less than 15 WU or Qp/Qs was greater than 1.25(Log rank test, P = 0.0001 and 0.001 respectively), but the actuarial survival at 10 and 15 yrs of the two groups reached no significantly difference when PVR was greater than 15 WU or Qp/Qs was less than 1.25 (Log rank test, P = 0.596 and 0.424 respectively).

Conclusion

The surgical closure therapy provides longer survival and much better life quality for the congenital systemic-to-pulmonary shunt and advanced pulmonary hypertension when it's PVR is less than 15 WU and/ or its Qp/Qs is greater than 1.25. Surgical criteria for congenital systemic-to-pulmonary shunt and advanced pulmonary hypertension should be revised as preoperative PVR less than 15 and Qp/Qs greater than 1.25.

Abbreviations

ACE	angiotensin-converting enzyme
ASD	atrial septal defect
APW	aorto-pulmonary windows
BSA	body surface area
CHD	congenital heart disease
CI	cardiac index
CO	cardiac output
CPB	cardiopulmonary bypass
CTR	cardiac to thoracic ratio
HR	hazard ratios
LVEF	left ventricular ejection fraction

mPAP	mean pulmonary artery pressure
NO	nitric oxide
OR	odds ratios
PAH	pulmonary arterial hypertension
PAP	pulmonary artery pressure
PCWP	pulmonary capillary wedge pressure
PDA	patent ductu aterisus
PVOD	pulmonary vascular occlusive disease
PVR	pulmonary vascular resistance
Qp/Qs	pulmonary to systemic flow ratio
6MWD	6 minute walk distance
SPAP	systolic pulmonary artery pressure
SPAP/SBP	pulmonary to systemic systolic artery pressure ratio
TPG	tran pulmonary pressure gradient
TTE	trans thoracic echocardiography
UVP	unidirectional valve patch
VSD	ventricular septal defect
WU	Wood Unit

There remains a striking paucity of management guidelines regarding operability in "borderline" patients with left to right shunts and PAH who usually present beyond infancy and early childhood [1,2]. With improving human development in many parts of the world, cardiac surgical centers now have to deal with a large population of untreated older children with CHD including several with "simple" shunt lesions and varying degrees of elevated PVR. There is therefore an urgent need to evolve management guidelines for these patients in whom assessment of operability remains a challenge [3]. From 1990, a nonrandomized study was commenced in Beijing Anzhen Hospital with an aim to investigate the relationship between the long-term survival of surgical treatment and preoperative pulmonary vascular resistance (PVR) and pulmonary to systemic flow ratio (Qp/Qs) in congenital systemic-to-pulmonary shunt and advanced PAH, and to put forward criteria for operability assessment.

Patients and Methods

The Institutional Review Board approved this study and written informed consent was obtained from each patient for the surgical procedure.

Patients

From February 1990 to July 2008, a total of 1572 patients of congenital systemic-to-pulmonary shunts and advanced PAH were recruited into and treated in Anzhen Hospital. For 1212 (77.1%) of these patients, complete preoperative homodynamic data were available from which to evaluate the association between early and late mortality and the calculated pulmonary homodynamic indices such as PVR, and Qp/Qs. Of the 1212 cases of patients, all were discussed preoperatively at a weekly multidisciplinary team meeting with pulmonary hypertension physicians, specialist radiologists and cardiac surgeons. For patients with PVR<10Wood Unit (WU), and /or Qp/Qs>1.50, the surgical team choose to close the defect; For patients with PVR≥20WU, and /or Qp/Qs≤1.0, the surgical team choose to recommend medical treatment; And for patients with PVR between 10 and 20 WU and Qp/Qs between 1.0 and 1.5, the operability was determined independently by the care providers in the cardiac surgical team of Beijing Anzhen Hospital after a comprehensive evaluation of the clinical information, history, physical examination, chest X-ray, arterial blood gas (ABG), ECG, echocardiography, and catheterization data, with the discretion of patients themselves and their family members, and the decision were made by consensus and conflicting opinions resolved by discussion between them. All data were entered prospectively into a dedicated surgical and pulmonary hypertension database, and based on whether or not undertaken a surgical closure procedure of the shunt, the patients were entered into 2 groups respectively; the non-surgical group (n=297 cases) and surgical group (n= 915). PAH is defined as a mean pulmonary artery pressure (mPAP) greater than 25 mm Hg at rest or 30 mm Hg with exercise and advanced PAH is further defined as a mPAP greater than 50 mm Hg, in line with the definition used by The American College of Chest Physicians [4,5]. Cardiac catheterizations were done under sedation and local anesthesia without intubation, and pulmonary artery pressure and mPAP and cardiac output (CO) were measured through a right heart catheterization on room air. Homodynamic parameters including right atrial, pulmonary artery, and pulmonary capillary wedge pressures were obtained according to standard clinical methods. CO was measured using a Fick's procedure (L/min). Body surface area was calculated from height and weight, cardiac index was calculated from CO and body surface area, and pulmonary homodynamic indices were calculated by means of the following equations: PVR (WU) = (mPAP - PCWP)/CO, where PCWP means precapillary wedge pressure. All patients were further submitted 10 min inhalation of 5 to 15 L/min facemask oxygen (100% oxygen), whereas 80% members in non-surgical group and 78% members in surgical group were also submitted to 10 min inhalation of 30 ppm of nitric oxide (NO) through a nasal cannula at the nares along with supplemental oxygen (O2) via face tent during right heart catheterization. A fall of PVR greater than 6 WU from baseline were assumed as positive reaction for oxygen or NO challenge. The mortality for the cardiac catheterization was 0%. Patients undergoing shunt closure that was combined with heart valve repair or replacement, or other surgical procedures were excluded. Patients with Down's syndrome were also excluded in the study population. Patients with residual heart defects after surgery, which may have had an impact on the severity of residual PAH were also excluded. Patients with heart defects that preclude an accurate calculation of PVR and Qp/Qs (branch pulmonary arterial stenosis, obstruction of isolated pulmonary veins, etc) were also excluded. The age when the diagnosis of a left to right shunt was established ranged from 12 months to 37 yrs old, and the age when the closure procedure was undertaken ranged from 13 months to 37 yrs old, and the interval between age at diagnosis and age at undertaken closure surgery was less than two weeks. The preoperative demographics and risk factors of the 1212 patients from the two groups are presented in Table 1.

End Point

The primary end point was defined as in-hospital death following surgery and late death. The second end point was defined as systolic pulmonary artery pressure (sPAP) as assessed through echocardiography and 6 minute walk distance (6MWD) at the follow-ups. The medical records of surviving patients were reviewed to determine whether care providers reported clinical evidence of right heart failure.

Table 1. Preoperative Baseline Demographic Variables and Risk Factors in Patients Receiving non-surgical Therapy and Patients Receiving surgical Therapy for the whole cohort of 1212 cases of patients

Patient Demographics and Preoperative Risk Factors	non-surgical group (Group A, n=297)	surgical group (Group B, n= 915)	P value
Age, yrs	25.8±8.5	18.4±8.1	0.0001
Age, yrs (interquarter percentile)	7.2-23.3	5.5-17.9	
Age older than 18 yrs old (%)	63.9	40.5	0.0001
Female (%)	35.5	34.7	0.709
Right heart failure (%)	25.5	20.2	0.005
Cyanosis			
Cyanosis at rest (%)	7.1	4.8	0.029
Cyanosis on exertion (%)	39.7	27.1	0.0001
Hemoglobin≥160g/L (%)	26.5	18.9	0.0001
Clubbing fingers and toes (%)	19.9	16.4	0.042
Systolic heart murmur≥II/6Grade (%)	37.8	88.5	0.0001
6MWD<500m (%)	27.5	16.1	0.0001
LVEF (%)	59.4±7.3	61.0±6.1	0.060
Bidirectional shunt on TTE (%)	68.3	45	0.0001
Severe tricuspid regurgitation (%)	36.8	27.4	0.0001
Right atrium pressure (mm Hg)	12.2±3.1	10.8±2.7	0.0001
PVR (Wood Unit)	18.9±6.5	12.05±6.8	0.0001
QP/Qs<1.25 (%)	41.6	25.3	0.0001
SPAP≥100mm Hg (%)	46.3	38.0	0.004
SPAP/SBP	0.97±0.18	0.87±0.15	0.000
mPAP (mm Hg)	81.5±17.2	69.7±15.2	0.040
SaO_2 (%)	88.8±5.5	92.5±4.2	0.0001
PaO_2<60 mm Hg (%)	22.8	12.9	0.0001
Hematoasthenia on chest X-ray (%)	23.6	18.9	0.010
CTR	0.63±0.064	0.62±0.069	0.097
Atrial fibrillation(n)	9	21	0.477
TRVAW(mm)	8.1±1.66	7.3±1.55	0.0001
CRBBB (%)	35.5	27.8	0.002
NYHA functional class≥III(%)	19.7	17.8	0.276
Shunt level			0.837
ASD (%)	11.3	10.8	

Patient Demographics and Preoperative Risk Factors	non-surgical group (Group A, n=297)	surgical group (Group B, n= 915)	P value
VSD (%)	58.2	58.9	
PDA (%)	11.1	19.5	
ASD+VSD (%)	7.0	7.0	
ASD+PDA (%)	2.2	2.2	
VSD+PDA (%)	7.9	7.0	
ASD+VSD+PDA (%)	1.2	1.5	
APW (%)	0.7	0.6	
Positive reaction to NO (%)	42.8	59.7	0.0001
Positive reaction to O_2 (%)	38.2	49.4	0.0001

6MWD=6 minute walk distance; LVEF=left ventricular ejection fraction; TTE=trans thoracic echocardiography; PVR= pulmonary vascular resistance; Qp/Qs= pulmonary to systemic flow ratio; SPAP=systolic pulmonary artery pressure; SPAP/SBP= pulmonary to systemic systolic artery pressure ratio, mPAP=mean pulmonary artery pressure; CTR=cardiac to thoracic ratio; CRBBB=complete right branch block, as defined the QRS interval longer than 0.12ms; TRAVW= the thickness of the right ventricular anterior wall, an indicator of right ventricular hypertrophy, were assessed through Tran thoracic echocardiography. VSD =ventricular septal defect; ASD=atrial septal defect; PDA=patent ductu aterisus; APW= aorto-pulmonary windows.

Therapeutic Regimen

All patients in surgical group were operated under general anesthesia and moderate hypothermic cardiopulmonary bypass (CPB) with cardiac arrest, and the shunts were closed through standard procedure. The non-surgical group and the surgical group during the follow-up were treated with a calcium channel blocker, and a cardiotonic glycoside, diuretic, anticoagulated with warfarin.

Follow up

Out of the 1212 patients, valid and complete follow up information were obtained in 1178 (97.2%) through outpatient department visiting. At one year following the discharge, all of these 1178 patients returned to Anzhen Hospital, for full review by the cardiac surgeon or pulmonary vascular disease physicians.

NYHA class, six-minute walk test, TTE and ECG data were recorded. These variables were again examined at every 12 month interval at their local PAH specialist centre. Long-term clinical outcome was assessed up to June 2008 by reviewing the medical files of their cardiologists or general practitioners, or both, when appropriate. Baseline demographics, procedural data, and perioperative outcomes were recorded. When a late death happened, the medical files must be reviewed by one of primary investigator of this study. A separate team of research assistants prospectively collected follow-up clinical data by telephone questionnaire after the patient was discharged from the hospital. The mean follow-up period was 97.2±57.36 months.

Statistical Analysis

All statistical analysis was performed with SAS for Windows Version 8.2 (SAS, Cary, NC). Categorical data are given as total numbers and relative frequencies. Continuous data are given as mean ± standard deviation. Comparisons between the two groups were made using the Mann–Whitney U-test, or the x^2 test as appropriate. The Kaplan–Meier survival curves were constructed to illustrate the actuarial survival. Comparisons of time-related data are made using Log-rank test. A p value of less than 0.05 was considered statistically significant. In an attempt to control for selection bias, propensity scores were estimated using unconditional logistic regression to determine the predicted probability of inclusion into the surgical group for each of the 1212 patients. First, to identify the character with which surgical closure of the shunts was liable to be selected, multivariate logistic regression was used. Of 28 defining baseline variables, 6 were not significant in the logistic regression analysis. These were sex, left ventricle ejection fraction, cardiac to thoracic ratio, the rhythm on ECG, the right ventricular hypertrophy sign on ECG, and NYHA functional class, and shunt level, and hemoptysis. Logistic regression analysis identified 8 variables as significant predictors of the surgical closure of the shunts. These 8 variables were PAP less than 110 mm Hg, and PVR less than 15 WU, and Qp/Qs greater than 1.25, and hemoglobin less than 160 g/L, a positive reaction to the pure oxygen inhalation in the right heart catheterization, and unidirectional systemic-to-pulmonary shunt on UCG, and a systolic heart murmur no less than Grade II out of 6 grade, and SaO_2 higher than 90%. Second, a propensity score was calculated for all 1212 patients using these significant regression coefficients. Each surgical closure patient was then closely matched with a non-surgical closure patient having the same or nearest propensity score (with the same propensity score±0.05, the matching approach is to attempt to match surgical and non-surgical subjects on the first five digits of the propensity score.). The matching was performed in the total population. This process successfully matched 245 patients who underwent surgical closure with 245 patients without surgical closure. The resulting 245 pairs of matched patients are the focus of the outcomes analysis in this study.

Preoperative variables, including the propensity score, were tested for a possible association with postoperative early mortality and late mortality. Variables were initially screened by univariate analysis. The univariate comparisons of outcomes were performed by means of the unpaired Student t test for numeric variables with normal distribution and by means of the Mann-Whitney U test for those without a normal distribution. Categorical variables were compared by means of the x^2 test as appropriate. Variables with a $P < 0.10$ at univariate analysis were then entered as independent variables in the stepwise logistic regression analyses and Cox proportional hazard analysis. Dependent variables were early mortality for the logistic regression analysis and late mortality for Cox proportional hazard analysis. All data were complete with the exception of reaction to NO inhalation during the right heart catheterization, which was only 80% complete. Only those variables significant at a 2-tailed nominal $P <0.05$ were retained within the logistic regression model and Cox proportional hazard analysis model. We get PVR≥15 WU, and Qp/Qs≤1.25, and hemoglobin ≥160g/L, and systemic $SaO_2 < 85\%$ remained in logistic regression equation, whereas PVR≥15 WU, and Qp/Qs≤1.25, and hemoglobin ≥160g/L remain in the Cox proportional hazard analysis equation. Odds ratios(OR) for logistic regression or hazard ratios(HR) for Cox proportional hazard analysis (Exp（B）) and corresponding 95% CI are reported with associated P values.

Results

The Results from the Whole Cohort of the 1212 Cases of Unmatched Patient

There happened 132 cases of PAH crisis during the peri operative period in the surgical group, out of which, 108 recovered through the PGE_1 or iloprost usage or NO inhalation and ventilation support during the ICU stay, and 24 died from the crisis. There happened 85 cases of acute right ventricular failure, out of which 80 recovered and 5 died due to the acute right heart failure. Thus there come up to a total of 29 peri operative deaths in the surgical group. Thus the surgical mortality for the 915 cases of the surgical group was 3.17%. With the follow-up of 97.2±57.36 months, there were 44 late deaths in the surgical group and 65 late deaths in the non-surgical group. Out of the total 109 cases of late death, 49 deaths were due to the refractory chronic right heart failure, 26 deaths were due to refractory arrhythmia, and 24 deaths were due to the PAH crisis, and 7 deaths were due to copious hemoptysis, 3 deaths were due to advanced lung infection.

Table 2. Preoperative Baseline Demographic Variables and Risk Factors of the Propensity-Matched Patients

Patient Demographics and Preoperative Risk Factors	non-surgical group (Group A, n=245)	surgical group (Group B, n= 245)	P value
Age, yrs	23.8±8.5	22.4±8.3	0.066
Age, yrs (interquarter percentile)	7.1-16.9	6.8-17.1	
Age older than 18 yrs old(n)	156	155	0.925
Female(n)	67	69	0.840
right heart failure(n)	62	61	0.917
Cyanosis			
Cyanosis at rest(n)	15	14	0.848
Cyanosis on exertion(n)	58	50	0.383
Hemoglobin(g/L)	158±25	157±24	0.652
Clubbing fingers and toes (n)	49	45	0.647
Systolic heart murmur≥II/6Grade (%)	85.7	86.5	0.7938
6MWD (meters)	545.9±78.0	556.5±65.8	0.105
LVEF (%)	59.2±7	60.2±7.2	0.087
Bidirectional shunt on TTE (n)	167	161	0.565
Severe tricuspid regurgitation(n)	90	88	0.851
Right atrium pressure (mm Hg)	11±3.2	11.5±2.9	0.4689
PVR (Wood Unit)	17.9±7.5	17.7±8.7	0.785
QP/QS	1.37±0.35	1.40±0.39	0.371
SPAP(mmHg)	106.3±18.6	108.0±15.9	0.277

Patient Demographics and Preoperative Risk Factors	non-surgical group (Group A, n=245)	surgical group (Group B, n= 245)	P value
SPAP/SBP	0.97±0.18	0.96±0.17	0.528
mPAP(mmHg)	76.5±17.2	75.8±16.4	0.645
SaO_2 (%)	86±6.3	85±5.5	0.062
PaO_2(mmHg)	72.8±13.6	74.2±15.5	0.288
Hematoasthenia on chest X-ray (n)	58	55	0.748
CTR	0.63±0.064	0.62±0.069	0.097
Atrial fibrillation(n)	7	5	0.400
TRVAW(mm)	7.6±1.71	7.5±1.62	0.5067
CRBBB	86	90	0.706
Hemoptysis(n)	10	8	0.631
NYHA functional class ≥III (n)	49	45	0.646
Shunt level(n)			0.930
ASD	28	30	
VSD	143	144	
PDA	27	24	
ASD+VSD	17	17	
ASD+PDA	5	6	
VSD+PDA	20	18	
ASD+VSD+PDA	3	5	
APW	2	1	
Positive reaction to NO(n)	115	101	0.197
Positive reaction to O_2(n)	95	104	0.880

6MWD=6 minute walk distance; LVEF=left ventricular ejection fraction; TTE=trans thoracic echocardiography; PVR= pulmonary vascular resistance; Qp/Qs= pulmonary to systemic flow ratio; SPAP=systolic pulmonary artery pressure; SPAP/SBP= pulmonary to systemic systolic artery pressure ratio, mPAP=mean pulmonary artery pressure; CTR=cardiac to thoracic ratio; CRBBB=complete right branch block, as defined the QRS interval longer than 0.12ms; TRAVW= the thickness of the right ventricular anterior wall, an indicator of right ventricular hypertrophy, were assessed through Tran thoracic echocardiography. VSD =ventricular septal defect; ASD=atrial septal defect; PDA=patent ductu aterisus; APW= aorto-pulmonary windows.

The Results from the 245 Propensity-Matched Pairs

All characteristics that differed significantly between two groups before matching became balanced (Table 2). There happened 65 cases of PAH crisis during the peri operative period in the surgical group, out of which, 53 recovered through the PGE₁ or iloprost usage or NO inhalation and ventilation support during the ICU stay, and 12 died from the crisis. There happened 45 cases of acute right ventricular failure, out of which 43 recovered and 2 died due to the acute right heart failure. Thus there come up to a total of 14 peri operative deaths in the surgical group. Thus the surgical mortality for the 245 cases of the propensity-matched surgical group was 5.71%. With the follow-up of 97.2±57.36 months, there were 13 late deaths in the surgical group and 37 late deaths in the non-surgical group. Out of the total 50 cases of late death, 18 deaths were due to the refractory chronic right heart failure, 11 deaths were due to refractory arrhythmia, and 15 deaths were due to the PAH crisis, and 5 were due to copious hemoptysis, 1 was due to advanced lung infection. 72 h post shunt closure procedure, the mPAP assessed through Swan-Ganz pulmonary artery catheter was 44.5±19.7 mm Hg for the PVR≤15 WU and 62.1±21.7 mm Hg for PVR > 15 WU (t=5.8043, P=0.0001). As shown in Figures 1, 2, 3 and 4 and Table 3, the Kaplan-Meier survival curves, with the PVR stratum at the level of 15 WU.m² and with the Qp/Qs stratum at the level of 1.25, were estimated to compare the long term actuarial survival between non-surgical group and surgical group in the 245 propensity score-matched pairs. the actuarial survival at 10 and 15 yrs of the surgical group was significantly higher than that of the non-surgical group with PVR less than 15 WU.m² or Qp/Qs larger than 1.25(Log rank test, $P = 0.0001$ and 0.001 respectively), but the actuarial survival at 10 and 15 yrs of the two groups reached no significantly difference with PVR greater than 15 WU.m² or Qp/Qs less than 1.25 (Log rank test, $P = 0.596$ and 0.424). The comparison of SPAP and 6MWD between the surgical and non-surgical group at follow-ups was shown at Table 4.

Table 3. The actuarial survival of the surgical and non-surgical for the 245 propensity matched pairs (%)

Stratum	Surgical group		Non-surgical group		P* value(χ^2)
	10yr	15yr	10yr	15yr	
PVR≥15 WU	83.90±4.5	73.90±9.3	83.8±4.1	62.5±7.3	0.596
PVR<15 WU	98.00±2.0	94.40±4.00	86.90±4.80	68.70±9.20	0.000
Qp/Qs<1.25	90.70±4.1	75.90±8.70	83.60±4.10	66.00±6.60	0.424
Qp/Qs≥1.25	97.90±2.1	94.00±4.30	87.2±4.47	69.9±8.80	0.001

* Log rank test of Kaplan-Meier survival curve between the surgical and non-surgical group.

The Management of Congenital Systemic-to-Pulmonary Shunt ... 91

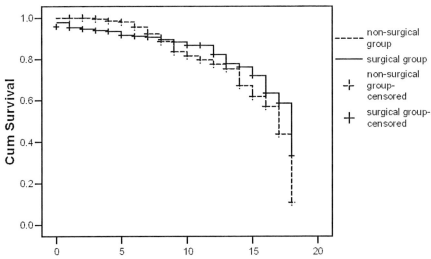

Figure 1. The Kaplan-Meier survival curve for the non-surgical therapy group and surgical therapy group when the PVR ≥ 15 Wood (survival years).

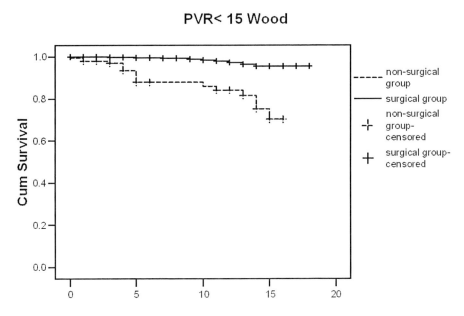

Figure 2. The Kaplan-Meier survival curve for the non-surgical therapy group and surgical therapy group when the PVR<15 Wood (survival years).

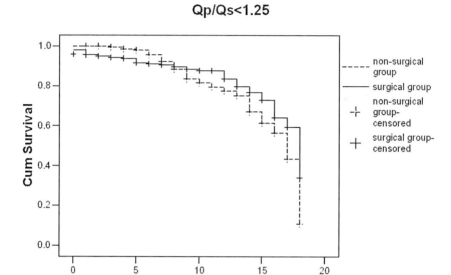

Figure 3. The Kaplan-Meier survival curve for the non-surgical therapy group and the surgical therapy group when the Qp/Qs<1.25 (survival years).

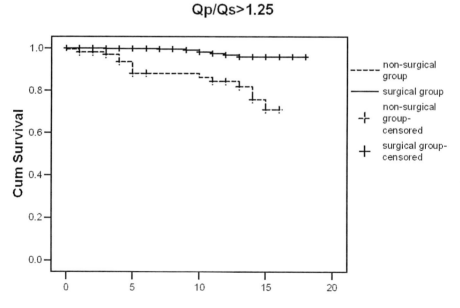

Figure 4. The Kaplan-meier survival curve for the non-surgical therapy group and the surgical therapy group when the Qp/Qs>1.24 (survival years).

Table 4. The comparison of SPAP and 6MWD between the surgical and non-surgical group at follow-ups

	sPAP(mm Hg)			6MWD (m)		
	Surgical Gr(n=218)	Non-surgical Gr(n=208)	P (t)	Surgical Gr (n=218)	Non-surgical Gr (n=208)	P (t)
PVR≤15 Wood	67.2±21.3(n=155)	101.7±17.1(n=65)	0.0001 (11.7119)	521.5±78.6(n=155)	443.9±65.2(n=65)	0.0001 (7.0146)
PVR>15 Wood	105.6±25.2(n=63)	109.7±21.1(n=143)	0.2280 (1.2091))	426±71.3(n=63)	418.9±82.0(n=143)	0.5524 (0.5951)
P (t)	0.0001 (11.5317)	0.0079 (2.983)		0.0001 (8.3468)	0.0314 (2.1670)	
Qp/Qs>1.25	70.2±17.8(n=152)	98.7±18.3(n=68)	0.0001 (10.8798)	535.7±74.5(n=152)	433.9±67.9(n=68)	0.0001 (9.6197)
Qp/Qs≤1.25	101.2±18.2(n=66)	106.7±19.1(n=140)	0.05179 (1.9575)	418±65.4(n=66)	409.9±82.0(n=140)	0.43529 (0.7818)
P (t)	0.0001 (11.7343)	0.0045 (2.8722)		0.0001 (11.1075)	0.0379 (2.0899)	

SPAP was estimated by Doppler using jet of ventricular septal defect and / or velocity of tricuspid and pulmonary regurgitation at follow-up, right atrium pressure were assumed as 10 mm Hg when making this calculations.

Table 5. The multivariate regression for the early death (binary logistic regression) and late death (Cox proportional hazard analysis) among Propensity-Matched Patients (n=245)

Events	Parameters	OR/HR (Exp(B))	95%CI of Exp(B)	B	SE of B	P value
Early death	PVR≥15 WU	3.756	1.092~12.913	1.323	0.630	0.036
	Qp/Qs≤1.25	6.233	1.981~19.610	1.830	0.585	0.002
	hemoglobin ≥ 160g/L	4.074	1.325~12.522	1.405	0.573	0.014
	systemic SaO$_2$ < 85%	3.96	1.093~14.493	1.378	0.658	0.036
Late death	PVR≥15 WU	11.628	4.274~31.25	2.451	0.511	0.000
	Qp/Qs≤1.25	4.831	1.473~15.873	1.577	0.607	0.009
	hemoglobin ≥ 160g/L	3.817	1.330~10.98	1.341	0.539	0.013

The Results of Multivariate Logistic Regression and Cox Proportional Hazard Analysis for the Propensity-matched Patients

As shown in Table 5, the multivariate logistic regression for the early death (binary logistic regression) revealed that PVR≥15 WU, and Qp/Qs≤1.25, and hemoglobin ≥160g/L, and systemic SaO_2 < 85% were the independent risk factors for the early death, and Cox proportional hazard analysis revealed that PVR≥15 WU, and Qp/Qs≤1.25, and hemoglobin ≥160g/L were the independent risk factors for the late death.

Discussion

Once irreversible PVOD is established, closure of a large shunt in a patient with advanced PVOD can be fatal either in the immediate postoperative period or on long-term follow-up. Therefore it is imperative to be certain of operability before referring such patients for surgery. In those with borderline changes in pulmonary vasculature, a comprehensive assessment must be made to test for operability. No technique is perfect for assessment of operability in a borderline case, and a comprehensive evaluation is necessary. A comprehensive evaluation should incorporate clinical information, chest X-ray, ECG, echocardiography, and catheterization data.

The technique most frequently used to evaluate the pulmonary vascular bed in congenital heart disease is cardiac catheterization [6,7,8]. PVR constitutes a key parameter in the pre-operative evaluation of the pulmonary vasculature. It is regarded as a measure of the functional state of the vascular bed [9], and the acute response of the vascular bed to vasodilators during cardiac catheterization is regarded as a measure of the reversibility of the disease process [10,11,12,13]. Supplemental oxygen may be used to decrease PVR and evaluate pulmonary vascular reactivity when PVR is excessively increased in room air alone. Nitric oxide may also be used to evaluate pulmonary vascular reactivity. However, it has to be acknowledged that the predictive value of acute testing of pulmonary vasoreactivity, with regard to the operability of the cardiac defect, the likelihood of a peri-operative pulmonary hypertensive crises, and persistent pulmonary hypertension following repair, has never been convincingly demonstrated in patients with congenital heart disease. Furthermore, recent observations in patients with advanced primary pulmonary hypertension, who did not respond to acute vasodilator testing, showed that long-term continuous epoprostenol therapy improved the clinical status and hemodynamic data [14,15]. Thus, vasodilator testing does not seem to add significantly to the baseline hemodynamic data and also introduces scope for errors in calculation. Although there is some data that suggests that the response to NO may aid in risk stratification and decision-making regarding timing of lung transplantation in patients with advanced PVOD [16,17], this cannot be extrapolated to this borderline situations where corrective surgery is being considered [18,19].

Many authors have used ratio of pulmonary-to-systemic vascular resistance. Unfortunately this ratio is also not ideal, as systemic resistance can be influenced by several variables. Higher preoperative pulmonary/systemic arterial pressure (Pp/Ps) and resistance (PVR/SVR) ratios are associated with more advanced stages of PVOD on lung biopsy and a higher incidence of early and late postoperative pulmonary hypertension [20].This relationship however is neither constant nor predictable and the degree of individual variability makes it difficult to apply a single cut-off to determine operability in these patients. Studies comparing hemodynamic data with lung biopsy findings as a "gold standard" are further limited by the questionable reliability of lung biopsy in determining operability in these situations [21].

Direct occlusion of a defect to eliminate the left to right shunt has been applied during hemodynamic evaluation to eliminate flow related PAH. Small case series have been published on the use of this potentially valuable technique in the assessment of operability particularly in adult patients with sizable PDA where complete occlusion of the duct is feasible [22]. Occlusion of a large ventricular septal defect is technically difficult. The PAP before and after occlusion are documented. A substantial fall in PAP may suggest operability [23]. The results may not be predictive of a long-term outcome.

Although determining operability is important in patients with left to right shunts who present late, until now, there remains a striking paucity of management guidelines regarding operability in "borderline" patients with left to right shunts and advanced PAH who usually present beyond infancy and early childhood. Early studies performed in the catheter laboratory were limited by small numbers and limited follow up and failed to establish clear cut-offs for operability [24]. With improving human development in many parts of the world, cardiac surgical centers now have to deal with a large population of untreated older children with CHD including several with "simple" shunt lesions and varying degrees of elevated PVR. There is therefore an urgent need to evolve management guidelines for these patients in whom assessment of operability remains a challenge. Efforts to evolve clear guidelines through careful prospective studies need to be undertaken as a number of patients with congenital heart defects in the developing world continue to present late with pulmonary hypertension.

There are many chaoses and heterogeneity existed in the existing literature for the guidelines of the operability assessment. A PVR index value of 6–8 WU (m^2) is widely accepted as a cut-off for operability in patients with large VSD or PDA [25]. These arbitrary boundaries are however constantly being challenged with the increasing use of postoperative pulmonary vasodilators and the advent of innovative surgical strategies [26]. Patients with atrial septal defects form a distinct subgroup and there remains much debate regarding the nature and underlying etiopathogenesis of PAH in this context [27]. Studies have demonstrated poorer outcomes with both medical and surgical therapy in patients with higher PVR. A total PVR greater than 15 Woods (m^2) units was associated with poor outcome following surgery in one retrospective analysis [28]. For patients with an atrial septal defect and PVOD with a predominant left-to-right shunt, some authors suggest the following approach to management: All patients with a total pulmonary resistance less than 10 WU/m^2 should proceed to operation; if the total PVR is 15 WU/ m^2 or greater then operation is not advised; if the total PVR is between 10 and 14 WU/ m^2, then operation should probably be performed, barring adverse findings with respect to systemic arterial oxygen saturation.

For the borderline patients, PVR and Qp/Qs would be the most important and subjective indices [29] but the criteria for admitting such patients of the borderline to surgical closure is not clear in term of numerical data of PVR and Qp/Qs in the lieu of contemporary medical progression. What should be the cut off level of PVR, and Qp/Qs to decide the surgical criteria for the patient of congenital systemic-to-pulmonary shunt and advanced PAH? From February 1990, a prospective but nonrandomized trial was commenced. After confirming the PVR and Qp/Qs as independent risk predictors for the long term survival, data were stratified according to the PVR and Qp/Qs level. This additional analysis revealed a significant difference of the survival between the surgical group vs. non-surgical group, but only at PCR≤15 WU or Qp/Qs>1.25. i.e. when the PVR was stratum at the of level of 15 WU, the long term actuarial survival rates diverged, i.e. when PVR <15 WU, the actuarial survival at 10 and 15 years in the surgical therapy group statistically were much higher than that of the non-surgical therapy group, but when PVR≥15 WU, the actuarial survival at 10 and 15 years were statistically the same between the two groups. Similar situation appeared when we stratum the Qp/Qs at the level of 1.25. To our further analysis of the life quality of these patients, it was also identified that when PVR≤15 Wood or Qp/Qs>1.25, the surgical treatment could provide a much better long term life quality in terms of 6MWD and lower SPAP as assessed through TTE. But when PVR >15WU or Qp/Qs≤1.25, this is not the case. This information reminded that the surgical criteria should be strictly controlled for congenital systemic-to-pulmonary shunts and advanced PAH, and we can revise the surgical criteria for this kind of patients from the old criteria. It is our suggestion that PVR ≥15 WU or/and Qp/Qs<1.25 could be chosen as the entry point for the contraindication criteria of surgical closure.

Study Limitation

This study is prospective but not randomized controlled trial, although being corrected through a propensity score matching, but may therefore involve too many confounding factors to show any clear relationship between the early and late prognosis and the PVR or Qp/Qs for the patients with congenital systemic-to-pulmonary shunts and advanced PAH. But the large number of patients that were enrolled for matching may get rid of some of the limitations.

Sources of Funding: This project was supported by of a grant (#81070041) from China Nature Science Foundation Committee.
Ethical approval: The Ethics Committee approved this retrospective study and written informed consent was obtained from each patient for the operation.
Competing interest: None declared.
The Conflict of Interest Disclosures: Hui-Li Gan now serves as an experienced surgeon in the phase III trials --the CHEST-1 and CHEST-2 study--on Riociguat, a novel drug that is currently in clinical development by Bayer Schering Pharma.

References

[1] Kannan BR, Sivasankaran S, Tharakan JA, Titus T, Ajith Kumar VK, Francis B, Krishnamoorthy KM, Harikrishnan S, Padmakumar R, Nair K. Long term outcome of patients operated for large ventricular septal defects

with increased pulmonary vascular resistance. *Indian Heart J* 2003; 55:161-166.

[2] Berger PMF. Possibilities and impossibilities in the evaluation of pulmonary vascular disease in congenital heart defects. *Eur Heart J* 2000; 21:17-27.

[3] Fried R, Falkovsky G, Newburger J, Gorchakova AI, Rabinovitch M, Gordonova MI, Fyler D, Reid L, Burakovsky V. Pulmonary arterial changes in patients with ventricular septal defects and severe pulmonary hypertension. *Pediatr Cardiol* 1986;7:147–154.

[4] Rubin LJ; American College of Chest Physicians. Diagnosis and management of pulmonary arterial hypertension: ACCP evidence-based clinical practice guidelines. *Chest.* 2004 Jul;126(1 Suppl):4S-6S.

[5] McLaughlin VV, Archer SL, Badesch DB, Barst RJ, Farber HW, Lindner JR, Mathier MA, McGoon MD, Park MH, Rosenson RS, Rubin LJ, Tapson VF, Varga J; American College of Cardiology Foundation Task Force on Expert Consensus Documents; American Heart Association; American College of Chest Physicians; American Thoracic Society, Inc; Pulmonary Hypertension Association. ACCF/AHA 2009 Expert Consensus Document on Pulmonary Hypertension: A Report of the American College of Cardiology Foundation Task Force on Clinical Expert Consensus Documents. *Circulation.* 2009 28;119(16):2250-94.

[6] Vargo TA. Cardiac catheterization. In: Garson Jr A, Bricker JT, Fisher DJ, Neish SR, eds. *The Science and Practice of Pediatric Cardiology.* Baltimore: Williams and Wilkins, 1998: 961–93.

[7] Bridges ND, Freed MD. Cardiac catheterization. In: Emmanouilides GC, Riemenschneider TA, Allen HD, Gutgesell HP, eds. *Moss and Adams Heart Disease in infants, Children and Adolescents, Including the Fetus and Young Adult,* 5th ed. Baltimore: Williams and Wilkins, 1995: 310–29.

[8] Lock JC, Keane JF, Fellows KE. *Diagnostic and interventional catheterization in congenital heart disease.* Boston: Martinus Nijhoff: 1987.

[9] Schostal SJ, Krovetz LJ, Rowe RD. An analysis of errors in conventional cardiac catheterization data. Am Heart J 1972; 83: 596.

[10] Berner M, Beghetti M, Spahr-Schopfer I, Oberhansli I, Friedli B. Inhaled nitric oxide to test the vasodilator capacity of the pulmonary vascular bed in children with long-standing pulmonary hypertension and congenital heart disease. *Am J Cardiol* 1996; 77: 532–5.

[11] Bush A, Busst C, Knight WB, Shinebourne EA. Modification of pulmonary hypertension secondary to congenital heart disease by prostacyclin therapy. *Am Rev Respir Dis* 1987; 136: 767–9.
[12] Bush A, Busst CM, Haworth SG, Hislop AA, Knight WB, Corrin B, Shinebourne EA. Correlations of lung morphology, pulmonary vascular resistance, and outcome in children with congenital heart disease. *Br Heart J* 1988; 59: 480–5.
[13] Rudolph AM. Cardiac catheterization and angiocardiography. In: Rudolph AM, ed. *Congenital Diseases of the Heart.* Chicago: Year Book Medical Publishers, Inc.1974: 49–167.
[14] Barst RJ, Rubin LJ, Long WA, McGoon MD, Rich S, Badesch DB, Groves BM, Tapson VF, Bourge RC, Brundage BH. A comparison of continuous intravenous epoprostenol (prostacyclin) with conventional therapy for primary pulmonary hypertension. *N Engl J Med* 1996; 334: 296–302.
[15] McLaughlin VV, Genthner DE, Panella MM, Rich S. Reduction in pulmonary vascular resistance with long-term epoprostenol (prostacyclin) therapy in primary pulmonary hypertension. *N Engl J Med* 1998; 338: 273–7.
[16] Post MC, Janssens S, Van de Werf, Budts W. Responsiveness to inhaled nitric oxide is a predictor of mid term survival in adult patients with congenital heart defects and pulmonary arterial hypertension. *Eur Heart J* 2004;25:1651–1656.
[17] Post MC, Janssens S, Van de Werf, Budts W. Responsiveness to inhaled nitric oxide is a predictor of mid term survival in adult patients with congenital heart defects and pulmonary arterial hypertension. *Eur Heart J* 2004;25:1651–1656.
[18] Fishman AP. Pulmonary hypertension: Beyond vasodilator therapy. *N Engl J Med* 1998; 338: 321–2.
[19] Balzer DT, Kort HW, Day RW, Corneli HM, Kovalchin JP, Cannon BC, Kaine SF, Ivy D, Webber SA, Rothman A, Ross RD, Aggarwal S, Takahashi M, Waldman JD. Inhaled nitric oxide as a preoperative test (INOP Test I): The INOP Test Study Group. *Circulation* 2002;106:76–81.
[20] Fried R, Falkovsky G, Newburger J, Gorchakova AI, Rabinovitch M, Gordonova MI, Fyler D, Reid L, Burakovsky V. Pulmonary arterial changes in patients with ventricular septal defects and severe pulmonary hypertension. *Pediatr Cardiol* 1986;7:147–154.

[21] Frescura C, Thiene G, Giulia Gagliardi M, Mazucco A, Pellegrino PA, Daliento L, Biscaglia S, Carminati M, Gallucci V. Is lung biopsy useful in surgical decision making in congenital heart disease? *Eur J Cardiothorac Surg* 1991;5: 118–122.
[22] Roy A, Juneja R, Saxena A. Use of Amplatzer ductal occluder to close severely hypertensive ducts: utility of transient balloon occlusion. *Indian Heart J* 2005;57:332–336.
[23] Yan C, Zhao S, Jiang S, Xu Z, Huang L, Zheng H, Ling J, Wang C, Wu W, Hu H, Zhang G, Ye Z, Wang H. Transcatheter closure of patent ductus arteriosus with severe pulmonary arterial hypertension in adults. *Heart* 2007;93:514–518.
[24] Momma K, Takao A, Ando M, Nakazawa M, Takamizawa K. Natural and post operative history of pulmonary vascular obstruction associated with ventricular septal defect. *Jpn Circ J* 1981;45:230–237.
[25] Yamaki S, Ogata H, Haneda K, Mohri H. Indications for open lung biopsy in patients with ventricular septal defect and/or patent ductus arteriosus and pulmonary hypertension. *Heart Vessels* 1990;5:166–171.
[26] Kannan BR, Sivasankaran S, Tharakan JA, Titus T, Ajith Kumar VK, Francis B, Krishnamoorthy KM, Harikrishnan S, Padmakumar R, Nair K. Long-term outcome of patients operated for large ventricular septal defects with increased pulmonary vascular resistance. *Indian Heart J* 2003;55:161–166.
[27] Therrien J, Rambihar S, Newman B, Siminovitch K, Langleben D, Webb G, Granton J. Eisenmenger syndrome and atrial septal defect: Nature or nurture? *Can J Cardiol* 2006;22:1133–1136.
[28] Steele PM, Fuster V, Cohen M, Ritter DG, Mc Goon DC. Isolated atrial septal defect with pulmonary vascular obstructive disease—Long term follow up and prediction of outcome after correction. *Circulation* 1987;76:1037–1042.
[29] Berman EB, Barst RJ. Eisenmenger's Syndrome: current management. *Prog Cardiovase Dis*. 2002; 45(2): 129-38.

In: Pulmonary Hypertension
Editor: Huili Gan
ISBN: 978-1-61470-556-7
© 2012 Nova Science Publishers, Inc.

Chapter IV

Systemic Inflammatory Response Syndrome Associated with Pulmonary Endarterectomy in Patients with Chronic Thromboembolic Pulmonary Hypertension

Pavel Maruna[1], Andrew A. Klein[2], Jan Kunstyr[3], Katerina M. Plocova[4], Frantisek Mlejnsky[4], David Ambroz[5], and Jaroslav Lindner[4]

[1]Department of Pathological Physiology of the First Faculty of Medicine, Charles University in Prague, Czech Republic
[2]Department of Anesthesia, Papworth Hospital, Cambridge, UK
[3]Department of Anesthesiology, Resuscitation and Intensive Medicine, General University Hospital and the First Faculty of Medicine, Charles University in Prague, Czech Republic
[4]2nd Surgical Department - Department of Cardiovascular Surgery, General University Hospital and the First Faculty of Medicine, Charles University in Prague, Czech Republic
[5]2nd Medical Department, General University Hospital and the First Faculty of Medicine, Charles University in Prague, Czech Republic

Abstract

Background

Pulmonary endarterectomy (PEA) is an effective treatment for chronic thromboembolic pulmonary hypertension (CTEPH). There are recent experimental findings suggesting the involvement of circulating cytokines such as interleukin-6 (IL-6), IL-8 and tumor necrosis factor-α (TNFα) in hemodynamic instability in the perioperative course of PEA. In a prospective study, the authors tested the hypothesis that elevated acute-phase reactants, induced by uncomplicated PEA, may influence haemodynamic parameters after PEA.

Material and Methods

92 patients (males/females 57/35, age 57 ± 8 yr.), treated with PEA using deep hypothermic circulatory arrest, were enrolled into the study. Plasma levels of IL-1β, IL-6, IL-8, TNFα, procalcitonin (PCT), C-reactive protein (CRP), ceruloplasmin and α_1-antitrypsin were measured repeatedly in arterial blood samples during the first 72 h after surgery.

Results

Mean duration of cardiopulmonary bypass (CPB) was 346.4 min.; mean circulatory arrest time was 37.6 min. All patients underwent satisfactory clearance of intra-arterial obstruction, and there were no intra-operative deaths. After PEA, there was considerable improvement in hemodynamic variables. In-hospital mortality for these patients was 4 / 92 (4.3 %).

PCT increased from baseline 0.22 ng/ml (0.16 – 0.29) (median (IQR)), reaching peak concentration 24 h after the end of surgery (2.04 ng/ml, 1.70 – 2.54). IL-6 rise was maximal at time of separation from CPB, 604.6 ng/l (517.6 – 698.2) with subsequent decline. TNFα rose from 17.4 ng/l (12.0 – 44.4) to maximum of 233.6 ng/l (138.2 – 434.0) over the same time course as IL-6. IL-8 and IL-1β peaked 12 h after the end of surgery. CRP, ceruloplasmin and α_1-antitrypsin showed prolonged elevation with a peak level 24 – 48 h after the end of surgery. Postoperative peak values of PCT and IL-6 correlated closely (r = 0.81, p = 0.004).

There was significant correlation between perioperative norepinephrine support and IL-6 plasma concentrations at separation from CPB (k = 0.754, p = 0.0071) and 12 h later (k = 0.813, p = 0.005). Similarly, duration of support with norepinephrine correlated positively with PCT at separation from CPB (k = 0.782, p = 0.0024) as well as with IL-8 at the same time (k = 0.715, p = 0.032). IL-6 plasma concentrations at separation from CPB correlated inversely with cardiac index (k = -0.653, p = 0.020).

Conclusion

PEA leads to pronounced activation of the cytokine network, PCT and acute-phase proteins. Hemodynamic instability after PEA is related to systemic inflammatory network activation. IL-6, IL-8 and PCT activation may be among the neurohumoral factors responsible for systemic vasoplegia and cardio-depression in CTEPH patients undergoing PEA.

Keywords: cardiopulmonary bypass, interleukin-6, interleukin-8, procalcitonin, pulmonary endarterectomy

Abbreviations

CI	Cardiac index
CPB	Cardiopulmonary bypass
CRP	C reactive protein
CTEPH	Chronic thromboembolic pulmonary hypertension
DHCA	Deep hypothermic circulatory arrest
ECC	Extracorporeal circulation
EF	Ejection fraction
IL	Interleukin
MAP	Mean artery pressure
MPAP	Mean pulmonary artery pressure
PCT	Procalcitonin
PEA	Pulmonary endarterectomy
PVR	Pulmonary vascular resistance
SIRS	Systemic inflammatory response syndrome
TNFα	Tumor necrosis factor-α

Introduction

Pulmonary endarterectomy (PEA) is the treatment of choice for patients with chronic thromboembolic pulmonary hypertension (CTEPH), whose prognosis would otherwise be very poor [Wittine and Auger 2010]. Untreated CTEPH is associated with a low five-year survival, ranging from 10 to 40%, dependent on the degree of elevation of the pulmonary artery pressure [Klok and Huisman 2010]. The goal of PEA is to improve pulmonary hemodynamics, exercise capacity, symptoms and survival. In many patients, hemodynamic parameters are normalized early after surgical intervention [Freed et al. 2011]. After successful endarterectomy, pulmonary artery pressure and pulmonary vascular resistance (PVR) fall and the cardiac output increases. At the present time, PEA is considered to be the only effective and potentially curative treatment for CTEPH. The procedure is associated with an improved six-year survival rate of 75% in appropriately selected patients [Ogino et al. 2006] and the outcome of PEA is better than that of pulmonary transplantation [Mayer and Klepetko 2006, Mayer 2010].

However the postoperative course after PEA is accompanied by a number of serious complications, which contribute to the relatively high rate of early postoperative mortality; this ranges from 5 - 23 %. Common causes of death are residual pulmonary hypertension, pulmonary reperfusion edema, right ventricular failure, and multi organ failure [Jamieson et al. 2003]. PEA is also associated with hemodynamic instability in the perioperative course. Profound systemic vasodilatation and cardiodepression frequently complicate postoperative management after PEA.

Additionally, patients undergoing PEA represent a major diagnostic challenge in terms of post-surgical inflammatory response. Due to the combination of local trauma, extracorporeal circulation (ECC), and pulmonary and myocardial reperfusion, PEA leads to substantial changes in the immune system that manifest as post-surgical systemic inflammatory response syndrome (SIRS). At the same time, the prolonged use of central venous catheters and inotropes are associated with a high risk of the development of nosocomial infection. There are recent reports suggesting the involvement of circulating mediators and cytokines such as interleukin-6 (IL-6), IL-8, tumor necrosis factor-α (TNFα) and procalcitonin (PCT) in systemic vasodilatation and cardiodepression [Comini et al. 2005, Giomarelli et al. 2003, Janssen et al. 2005, Wei et al. 2003].

In this prospective study, the authors tested the hypothesis that elevated acute phase reactants, induced by uncomplicated PEA may influence hemodynamic parameters and the difficulty of controlling arterial blood pressure after PEA. The selection of measured inflammatory parameters came from a previous pilot study evaluating postoperative SIRS in 36 patients undergoing uncomplicated PEA [Lindner et al. 2009]. In agreement with published experimental findings [Ishida et al. 2007, Parolari et al. 2007], preliminary clinical results supported the role of IL-6 and IL-8 in post-operative hemodynamic instability.

Material and Methods

The study was approved by the Research Ethics Committee of the 1St Faculty of Medicine, Charles University and General Teaching Hospital in Prague. The ethical committee of the institution approved the study protocol and written informed consent was obtained. Patients with CTEPH scheduled for isolated PEA surgery between January 2007 and December 2010 were included. Exclusion criteria were PEA combined with another procedure and proven local or systemic infection defined according to guidelines of the Center for Disease Control and Prevention [Horan and Gaynes 2004].

Surgical Procedure

All patients underwent PEA via median sternotomy. Cardiopulmonary bypass (CPB) was established after cannulation of the ascending aorta and the inferior and superior vena cava. The CPB circuit consisted of roller pumps (Stoeckert, Germany), standard tubing and a membrane oxygenator (Medos, Germany). Deep hypothermic circulatory arrest (DHCA, 18-20 ^{0}C) was used (limited to 20 minute episodes), to ensure optimum operating conditions and facilitate accurate endarterectomy. Endarterectomy was started with dissection of the right pulmonary artery and continued into the segmental branches. Subsequently, arteriotomy on of the left PA was carried out and continued down the arterial tree. After completion of endarterectomy on the both sides and closure of the PA,controlled rewarming was commenced. Weaning from CPB commenced with pressure control ventilation of the lungs with positive end-expiratory pressure, atrio-ventricular epicardial stimulation, stepwise increased filling of the right heart and reduction of pump flow together with low doses of norepinephrine targeted to reach a mean pulmonary artery pressure (MPAP) less than 20 mmHg and mean arterial pressure over 70 mmHg. Dobutamine (Dobutrex, Lily, Germany) was administered only if inotropic support was needed during or after weaning of CPB. Cardiac function was evaluated echocardiographically and dobutamine was administered in doses of 5-10 µg/kg/min.

Anesthetic Management

All patients were premedicated with 0.1 mg·kg^{-1} of diazepam (Diazepam, Zentiva, SR) orally. After transfer to the operating room, patients were administered total intravenous anesthesia, standard for this procedure in our institution. This consists of sufentanil (Sufenta, Janssen, Belgium) 0.5 µg·kg^{-1}, midazolam (Dormicum, Roche, CR) 3-5 mg, propofol (Diprivan, AstraZeneca, UK) 1 mg·kg^{-1} and rocuronium (Esmeron, Schering-Plough, France) 0.6 mg·kg^{-1} intravenously. Anesthesia was maintained with a continuous infusion of propofol and sufentanil with BIS targeted at 40 to 50. Further incremental doses of rocuronium 5-10 mg were administered if interference with the ventilator was noted.

Hemodynamic Status

Hemodynamic monitoring included central venous catheter, femoral artery catheter, a surgically placed left atrial catheter and flow–directed Swan-Ganz catheter. The basic hemodynamic parameters followed were: MPAP, cardiac index (CI), PVR, and ejection fraction (EF).

Cytokines, PCT and acute-phase proteins analysis

Arterial blood samples were drawn from the femoral artery catheter before incision, after sternotomy, after the last period of DHCA, after separation from CPB, and 12, 18, 24, 36 and 48 h after surgery. 5 ml of arterial blood was taken into a vacutainer tube and centrifuged at 5000 rpm for 15 min. Plasma was stored at -80°C. Plasma levels of TNFα, IL-1β, IL-6, and IL-8 (ELISA, Immunotech, Paris, France), PCT, C-reactive protein (CRP) (Kryptor - TRACE, BRAHMS

AG, Hennigsdorf, Germany), ceruloplasmin and α1-antitrypsin (nephelometry, BRAHMS AG, Hennigsdorf, Germany) were measured in duplicates. The intra- and inter- assay coefficients of variation were below 5%.

Statistical Analysis

Data was analyzed using the Statistical Package for Social Sciences, version 18.0 for Windows (SPSS Inc., Chicago, USA). The power calculation was undertaken using Sample Power 2.0; the sample size calculation was based on a two-sided two-sample testing, a significance level of 0.05 and a power of 90% and 90 patients were found to be required. Distribution of data was examined using the Kolmogorov-Smirnov normality test to determine subsequent use of tests for statistical comparison. As variables were not normally distributed, the data were reported as median and interquartile range. The Mann-Whitney test was applied for data comparison between groups. Bonferroni correction was used to analyze simultaneous measurement at different time points.

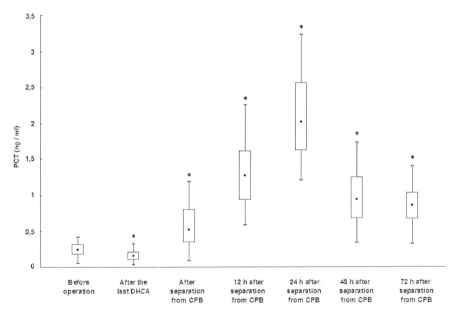

* ... Statistically significant differences comparing to preoperative values, $p < 0.05$.

Figure 1. Perioperative dynamics of PCT in patients undergoing uncomplicated PEA. Median values and interquartile range are described.

Table 1. Demographic characteristics and hemodynamic status of PEA patients (n = 92)

Number of males (%)		57 (62 %)	
Age (yr.)		57.4 (8.4)	
Ejection fraction (%)	preoperatively	60.2 (8.9)	
Mean pulmonary artery pressure (mm Hg)	preoperatively	55.8 (8.1)	$p = 0.00032$
	postoperatively	24.6 (7.1)	
Cardiac index (l.min^{-1}m^{-2})	preoperatively	1.9 (0.4)	$p = 0.00020$
	postoperatively	3.0 (0.5)	
Pulmonary vascular resistance (dynes.s.cm^{-5})	preoperatively	1112.4 (310.7)	$p = 0.000017$
	postoperatively	206.4 (96.0)	

Variables are absolute number or mean (standard deviation).
Postoperative data are given 24 hours after admission to intensive care unit.

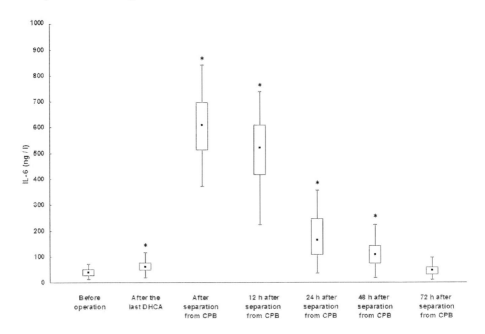

* ... Statistically significant differences comparing to preoperative values, $p < 0.05$.

Figure 2. Perioperative dynamics of IL-6 in patients undergoing uncomplicated PEA. Median values and interquartile range are described.

Results

92 patients were enrolled during the 4 years of the trial (Table 1). All patients underwent satisfactory clearance of intra-arterial obstruction, and there were no intra-operative deaths. No patients required allogenic blood transfusion. Hemodynamic and clinical improvements after PEA were very convincing. MPAP and PVR decreased significantly and CI was increased within the first 24 h.

Transient initial decline of IL-6, IL-8 and PCT (minimum 3 h after sternotomy) correlated significantly with decreased hematocrit during hemodilution ($r = 0.863$, $p = 0.0019$ for IL-6; $r = 0.827$, $p = 0.0044$ for IL-8; $r = 0.641$, $p = 0.012$ for PCT). PCT increased from initial levels of 0.22 ng/ml (0.16 – 0.29) (mean (IQR)), reaching peak concentrations 24 h after surgery (2.04 ng/ml, 1.70 – 2.54) (Figure 1). Preoperative IL-6 plasma concentrations were 19.3 ng/l (10.4 – 31.6). IL-6 rise was maximal at the time of separation from CPB, 604.6 ng/l (517.6 – 698.2), with subsequent decline (Figure 2). TNFα rose from 17.4 ng/l (12.0 – 44.4) to a maximum of 233.6 ng/l (138.2 – 434.0) at the same time as IL-6 maximum. IL-8 (initial concentrations 86.1 ng/l (44.2 – 137.6)) peaked 12 h after surgery at 441.6 ng/l (237.7 – 638.1). The same time course was shown for IL-1β, starting from preoperative levels 8.3 ng /l (2.9 – 11.4) to maximum concentration at the time of separation from CPB (53.1 ng/l, 29.0 – 76.2). CRP, ceruloplasmin and $α_1$-antitrypsin showed prolonged elevation with a peak level 24 – 48 h after surgery. Postoperative peak values of PCT and IL-6 correlated closely ($r = 0.831$, $p = 0.004$).

The patients with preoperative functional classification NYHA IV had higher levels of TNFα and IL-6 preoperatively compared with patients with NYHA III. This difference was statistically significant for IL-6 ($p = 0.036$). No correlation was revealed between preoperative hemodynamic variables (MPAP, CI, PVR, EF) and preoperative plasma levels of measured cytokines, PCT and acute-phase proteins.

There was significant correlation between perioperative norepinephrine support and IL-6 plasma concentration at the time of separation from CPB ($k = 0.754$, $p = 0.0071$) and 12 h later ($k = 0.813$, $p = 0.005$) (Figure 3). Similarly, duration of support with norepinephrine correlated positively with PCT at separation from CPB ($k = 0.782$, $p = 0.0024$) as well as with IL-8 at the same time ($k = 0.715$, $p = 0.032$). IL-6 plasma concentration at the time of separation from CPB correlated inversely with CI ($k = -0.653$, $p = 0.020$). Individual maximum doses of norepinephrine during PEA were compared with cytokine plasma levels during the same period, however there was no statistical significance for any of the inflammatory parameters.

IL-6 plasma concentrations at the time of separation from CPB correlated inversely with CI (k = -0.693, p = 0.0144). No significant relationship was found between postoperative cytokine levels and MPAP or PVR.

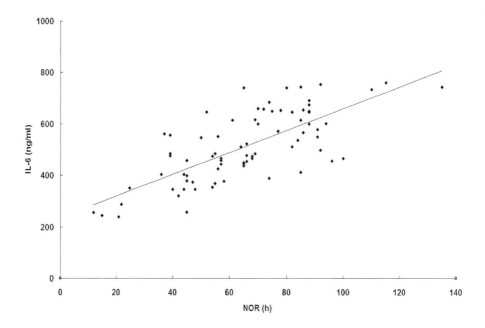

Figure 3. Correlation of IL-6 arterial concentration at 12 h after the separation from CPB and the time of norepinephrine support, k = 0.754, p = 0.0071.

Conclusion

In this study, uncomplicated PEA induced a postoperative cytokine network response with a subsequent increase in serum PCT and acute phase protein levels. Levels of proinflammatory cytokines IL-1β, IL-6 and TNFα culminated at the time of separation from CPB, while IL-8 reached maximum concentrations 12 h after surgery. Peak PCT levels were demonstrated 24 h postoperatively. Transient initial decline of IL-6, IL-8 and PCT can be explained mostly by hemodilution. We suspect that hemofiltration used for hemoconcentration before weaning from CPB may also lead to decreased levels of cytokines in the perioperative phase.

Hemodynamic status after PEA was related to the cytokine inflammatory network. Higher concentrations of IL-6 were associated with lower CI in perioperative period, and patients with a higher demand for catecholamine support in the perioperative period showed significantly higher plasma concentrations of IL-6, IL-8 and PCT.

TNFα, IL-1β and IL-6 are major proinflammatory cytokines involved in the acute inflammatory response as well as in the pathogenesis and outcome of SIRS, sepsis, and septic shock [Maruna et al. 2011, Sutherland et al. 2005]. Increased levels of cytokines have been reported in patients undergoing on-pump coronary artery bypass surgery compared to those without CPB [Nesher et al. 2006]. However, Franke et al. [2005] showed that CPB is far less important in this context and they concluded that surgical trauma and reperfusion injury of the lung parenchyma appears to represent the predominant factor resulting in immunological changes after cardiac surgery. Other factors may influence cytokine production after cardiac surgery, too. Continued ventilation during CPB resulted in lesser pro-inflammatory cytokine response than CPB without ventilation [Ng et al. 2008].

The kinetics of the main proinflammatory cytokines after PEA was described firstly by Langer et al. [2004]. In a relatively small group of 14 patients, they revealed a positive correlation between maximum vasopressor support and peak levels of IL-6. In our study, the duration of catecholamine support was demonstrated as a better parameter reflecting hemodynamic instability than maximum doses of norepinephrine.

Hemodynamic instability is common after PEA and the management of patients differs from the management of patients after other cardiosurgical procedures. A borderline CI with low preload is well tolerated and low MPAP is mandatory in order to prevent detrimental reperfusion injury; inotropic agents are indicated only if clinical and echocardiographic signs of cardiac failure occur.

This study has documented that the time of post-surgery catecholamine support was related to IL-6 and IL-8 levels. A higher demand for norepinephrine support in the perioperative period is a marker of hemodynamic instability following PEA. The dose of norepinephrine is related to mean arterial pressure and its prolonged administration is necessary in persisting vasoplegia with hypotension. Therefore we assume that norepinephrine consumption may well reflect the hemodynamic status of the patient in this situation. Our results are in agreement with the explanation that IL-6 and IL-8 activation may be among the neurohumoral factors responsible for the systemic vasoplegia and cardio-depressive effect in CTEPH patients undergoing PEA.

Cardiac surgery leads to a more pronounced activation of cytokines than other surgical procedures [Chachkhiani et al. 2005]. This cytokine 'burst' mediates a systemic response by the body's inflammatory system, known as the systemic inflammatory response syndrome. Martínes-Rosaz et al. [2006] reviewed recent papers supporting the idea of a cardioprotective role for an early inflammatory response. They postulated that TNFα and IL-6 negative inotropic effects could represent to a certain extent a non-specific adaptive response to delimit the ischemic injury and to decrease myocardial energy demand. The potential physiological importance of cytokine-mediated cardio depressive effects is not yet clear.

Maximum PCT values around 2.0 ng/ml as documented in our patients are in agreement with other authors (range from 0.5 to 7.0 ng/ml) [Baykut et al. 2000, Celebi et al. 2006, Franke et al. 2005, Michalik et al. 2006]. PCT, a protein of 116 amino-acids with molecular weight of 13 kD, was discovered 35 years ago as a prohormone of calcitonin produced by C-cells of the thyroid gland. Since 1993 when its' elevated level was found in patients with bacterial infection [Assicot et al. 1993], PCT became an important marker in the detection and differential diagnostics of inflammatory states. The highest plasma levels of PCT are achieved in acute bacterial infections and sepsis. Plasma levels are enhanced by the presence of a systemic inflammatory response. Local bacterial infections as well as abscesses do not raise plasma PCT significantly [Maruna et al. 2000].

Several factors may influence the evolution of serum PCT levels after cardiac surgery in the absence of postoperative complications. The increase of PCT seems to be dependent on the surgical procedure, with more invasive procedures associated with higher PCT levels [Sponholz et al. 2006]. The source of PCT production in these conditions can be explained by non-specific cytokine liberation from injured tissue [Kerbaul et al. 2002]. The subsequent decline of PCT levels to normal within a few days after surgery after uncomplicated surgery corresponds to the half-life of PCT (18 to 24 h) in the absence of a further insult that may induce more PCT production [Arkader et al. 2004].

To date, all of the physio-pharmacological studies that have been performed to evaluate the physiological role of PCT in inflammation have indicated potentially harmful effects. PCT interacts with immune cells in a feedback manner, and its overproduction may further augment the local levels of pro-inflammatory cytokines. In vitro studies did not document a direct influence of PCT on hemodynamic parameters. However, Hoffmann et al. (2002) showed that the addition of PCT acts as a potent amplifier of the inducible nitric oxide synthase gene expression in vitro if vascular smooth muscle cells were previously primed with pro-inflammatory stimulus. Increased levels of nitric oxide as a potent vasodilator occur in sepsis, and high values are found in patients with complicating hypotension [Mitaka et al. 2003].

In summary, PEA leads to a pronounced activation of the cytokine network, PCT and acute phase proteins. Hemodynamic instability after PEA is related to enhanced systemic inflammatory network activation. IL-6, IL-8, and possible PCT activation may be among the neurohumoral factors responsible for the systemic vasoplegia and cardio-depressive effect in CTEPH patients undergoing PEA.

Acknowledgment

The study was supported with a grant IGA NT11210-4/2010 of the Ministry of Health, Czech Republic.

References

Arkader R, Troster EJ, Abellan DM, Lopes MR, Júnior RR, Carcillo JA, Okay TS: Procalcitonin and C-reactive protein kinetics in postoperative pediatric cardiac surgical patients. *J Cardiothorac Vasc Anesth,* 2004, 18, 160-165.

Assicot M, Gendrel D, Carsin H, Raymond J, Guilbaud J, Bohuon C: High serum procalcitonin concentrations in patients with sepsis and infection. *Lancet,* 1993, 341, 515-518.

Baykut D, Schulte-Herbrüggen J, Krian A: The value of procalcitonin as an infection marker in cardiac surgery. *Eur J Med Res,* 2000, 5, 530-536.

Celebi S, Koner O, Menda F, Balci H, Hatemi A, Korkut K, Esen F: Procalcitonin kinetics in pediatric patients with systemic inflammatory response after open heart surgery. *Intensive Care Med,* 2006, 32, 881-887.

Comini L, Pasini E, Bachetti T, Dreano M, Garotta G, Ferrari R: Acute haemodynamic effects of IL-6 treatment in vivo: involvement of vagus nerve in NO-mediated negative inotropism. *Cytokine,* 2005, 30, 236-242.

Franke A, Lante W, Fackeldey V, Becker HP, Kurig E, Zoller LG, Weinhold C, Markewitz A: Pro-inflammatory cytokines after different kinds of cardio-thoracic surgical procedures: is what we see what we know? *Eur J Cardiothorac Surg,* 2005, 28, 569-575.

Freed DH, Thomson BM, Berman M, Tsui SS, Dunning J, Sheares KK, Pepke-Zaba J, Jenkins DP: Survival after pulmonary thromboendarterectomy: Effect of residual pulmonary hypertension. *J Thorac Cardiovasc Surg*, 2011, 141, 383-387.

Giomarelli P, Scolletta S, Borrelli E, Biagioli B: Myocardial and lung injury after cardiopulmonary bypass: role of interleukin (IL)-10. *Ann Thorac Surg*, 2003, 76, 117-123.

Hoffmann G, Czechowski M, Schloesser M, Schobersberger W: Procalcitonin amplifies inducible nitric oxide synthase gene expression and nitric oxide production in vascular smooth muscle cells. *Crit Care Med*, 2002, 30, 2091–2095.

Horan TC, Gaynes RP: Surveillance of nosocomial infections. Appendix A. CDC definitions of nosocomial infections. In Mayahall CG (3rd ed): *Hospital Epidemiology and Infection Control*. Philadelphia: Lippincot Williams and Wilkins, 2004, pp. 1659–702.

Chachkhiani I, Gurlich R, Maruna P, Frasko R, Lindner J: The postoperative stress response and its reflection in cytokine network and leptin plasma levels. *Physiol Res*, 2005, 54, 279-285.

Ishida K, Masuda M: Thromboendarterectomy for severe chronic thromboembolic pulmonary hypertension, *Asian Cardiovasc Thorac Ann*, 2007, 15, 229-233.

Jamieson SW, Kapelanski DP, Sakakibara N, Manecke GR,Thistlethwaite PA, Kerr KM,Channick RN,Fedullo PF,Auger WR. Pulmonary endarterectomy: Experience and lesson learned in 1,500 cases. *Ann Thorac Surg*, 2003, 76, 1457-1464.

Janssen SPM, Gayan-Ramirez G, Van Den Bergh A, Herijgers P, Maes K, Verbeken E, Decramer M: Interleukin-6 causes myocardial failure and skeletal muscle atrophy in rats. *Circulation*, 2005, 111, 996-1005.

Kerbaul F, Guidon C, Lejeune PJ, Mollo M, Mesana T, Gouin F: Hyperprocalcitoninemia is related to noninfectious postoperative systemic inflammatory distress syndrome associated with cardiovascular dysfunction after coronary artery bypass graft surgery. *J Cardiothorac Vasc Anesth*, 2002, 16, 47-53.

Klok FA, Huisman MV: Epidemiology and management of chronic thromboembolic pulmonary hypertension. *Neth J Med*, 2010, 68, 347-351.

Langer F, Schramm R, Bauer M, Tscholl D, Kunihara T, Schafers HJ. Cytokine response to pulmonary thromboendarterectomy. *Chest*, 2004, 126, 135-141.

Lindner J, Maruna P, Kunstyr J, Jansa P, Gürlich R, Kubzová K, Zakharchenko M, Linhart A: Hemodynamic instability after pulmonary endarterectomy for

chronic tromboembolic pulmonary hypertension correlates with cytokine network hyperstimulation. *Eur Surg Res,* 2009, 43, 39-46.
Martínez Rosas M: Cardiac remodeling and inflammation. *Arch Cardiol Mex,* 2006, 76, S58-S66.
Maruna P, Nedelnikova K, Gürlich R: Physiology and genetics of procalcitonin. *Physiol Res,* 2000, 49, S57-S61.
Maruna P: Prokalcitonin. *Triton,* Prague, 2003.
Maruna P, Kunstyr J, Plocova KM, Mlejnsky F, Hubacek JA, Klein A, Lindner J: Predictors of infection after pulmonary endarterectomy for thromboembolic pulmonary hypertension. *Eur J Cardio-Thorac,* 2011, 39, 195-200.
Mayer E, Klepetko W. Techniques and outcomes of pulmonary endarterectomy for chronic thromboembolic pulmonary hypertension. *Proc Am Thorac Soc,* 2006, 3, 589-593.
Mayer E: Surgical and post-operative treatment of chronic thromboembolic pulmonary hypertension. *Eur Respir Rev,* 2010, 19, 64-67.
Mehta S, Helmersen D, Provencher S, Hirani N, Rubens FD, De Perrot M, et al.: Diagnostic evaluation and management of chronic thromboembolic pulmonary hypertension: A clinical practice guideline. *Can Respir J,* 2010, 17, 301-334.
Michalik DE, Duncan BW, Mee RB, Worley S, Goldfarb J, Danziger-Isakov LA, Davis SJ, Harrison AM, Appachi E, Sabella C: Quantitative analysis of procalcitonin after pediatric cardiothoracic surgery. *Cardiol Young,* 2006, 16, 48-53.
Mitaka C, Hirata Y, Yokoyama K, Wakimoto H, Hirokawa M, Nosaka T, Imai T: Relationships of circulating nitrite/nitrate levels to severity and multiple organ dysfunction syndrome in systemic inflammatory response syndrome. *Shock,* 2003, 19, 305–309.
Nesher N, Frolkis I, Vardi M, Sheinberg N, Bakir I, Caselman F, Pevni D, Ben-Gal Y, Sharony R, Bolotin G, Loberman D, Uretzky G, Weinbroum AA: Higher levels of serum cytokines and myocardial tissue markers during on-pump versus off-pump coronary artery bypass surgery. *J Card Surg,* 2006, 21, 395-402.
Ng CS, Arifi AA, Wan S, Ho AM, Wan IY, Wong EM, Yim AP: Ventilation during cardiopulmonary bypass: impact on cytokine response and cardiopulmonary function. *Ann Thorac Surg,* 2008, 85, 154-162.
Ogino H, Ando M, Matsuda H, Minatoya K, Sasaki H, Nakanishi N, Kyotani S, Imanaka H, Kitamura S: Japanese single-center experience of surgery for

chronic thromboembolic pulmonary hypertension. *Ann Thorac Surg,* 2006, 82, 630-636.

Parolari A, Camera M, Alamanni F, Naliato M, Polvani GL, Agrifoglio M, Brambilla M, Biancardi C, Mussoni L, Biglioli P, Tremoli E: Systemic inflammation after on-pump and off-pump coronary bypass surgery: a one-month follow-up. *Ann Thorac Surg,* 2007, 84, 823-828.

Sponholz C, Sakr Y, Reinhart K, Brunkhorst F: Diagnostic value and prognostic implications of serum procalcitonin after cardiac surgery: a systematic review of the literature. *Crit Care,* 2006, 10, R145.

Sutherland AM, Walley KR, Manocha S, Russell JA: The association of interleukin 6 haplotype clades with mortality in critically ill adults. *Arch Intern Med,* 2005, 165, 75-82.

Wei M, Kuukasjärvi P, Laurikka J, Kaukinen S, Honkonen EL, Metsänoja R, Tarkka M: Relation of cytokines to vasodilation after coronary artery bypass grafting. *World J Surg,* 2003, 27, 1093-1098.

Wittine LM, Auger WR: Chronic thromboembolic pulmonary hypertension. *Curr Treat Options Cardiovasc Med,* 2010, 12, 131-141.

Reviewed by: Pavel Jansa, M.D., 2nd Medical Department – Clinical Department of Cardiology and Angiology of the First Faculty of Medicine, Prague, Czech Republic.

In: Pulmonary Hypertension
Editor: Huili Gan

ISBN: 978-1-61470-556-7
© 2012 Nova Science Publishers, Inc.

Chapter V

Liver Transplantation and Pulmonary Hypertension

Michael Ramsay[*]
Chairman Department of Anesthesiology, Baylor University Medical Center
Dallas Texas, US

Abstract

Portopulmonary hypertension is found in 5-6% of patients with portal hypertension. This may or may not be associated with liver cirrhosis. If cirrhosis is present the severity of the liver cirrhosis does not correlate with the degree of pulmonary hypertension. The diagnosis of portopulmonary hypertension includes a mean pulmonary artery pressure of greater than 25 mm Hg at rest and a pulmonary vascular resistance of greater than 240 dynes.s.cm^{-5} and the presence of portal hypertension. Approximately 20% of patients with liver cirrhosis presenting for liver transplantation will have increased pulmonary artery pressures, but in the majority of patients this is the result of intravascular volume overload, together with a high flow state that is typically seen in patients with liver cirrhosis and this may be further affected by the presence of a cirrhotic cardiomyopathy. However the key differentiator of these causes of pulmonary hypertension from true

---

[*] Tel: +1-214-820-3296; E-mail: docram@baylorhealth.edu

portopulmonary hypertension is that in this group the pulmonary vascular resistance is normal or low.

The etiology of portopulmonary hypertension is not well understood. Initially endothelial dysfunction in the pulmonary arterioles may occur as the result of sheer stress forces from the high velocity circulation and the toxic effects of inflammatory molecules that are either not cleared by the liver or are released by the diseased liver.

The clinical symptoms may be minimal in the early phases of the disease but as it progresses shortness of breath, chest pain, fatigue, palpitations and syncope may present. However these symptoms are not distinct from those of progressive liver disease, therefore all liver transplant candidates should be screened for portopulmonary hypertension. The current screening tool is the transthoracic Doppler echocardiogram. If the right ventricular systolic pressure is 50 mm Hg. or greater a right heart catheterization should be performed and the pulmonary vascular resistance calculated. Once the diagnosis of portopulmonary hypertension has been made a careful assessment of right ventricular function is required by echocardiography. Liver transplantation will treat many of these patients but not all, and it cannot be predicted which patients will respond to transplantation. The risks of liver transplantation increase with the severity of the pulmonary hypertension and those patients with evidence of right heart dysfunction should undergo pulmonary vasodilator therapy prior to consideration for transplant.

Introduction

Portal hypertension with and without liver cirrhosis has been associated with pulmonary complications [1]. One of these complications is pulmonary artery hypertension and when this is associated with portal hypertension it is termed portopulmonary hypertension (POPH). This is a very serious complication for the patient, as the right heart ventricle (RV) is well designed to pump volume but only at low pressures and low after load. The RV does not have the muscle power to handle the increased workload if a significant increase in pulmonary vascular resistance (PVR) occurs unless this increase in after load is gradual and hypertrophy of the ventricle muscle can take place. If this increase in RV wall strength does not occur the right heart will become dilated and dysfunctional resulting in venous congestion of the liver. Eventually as the POPH progresses right heart failure will occur and eventual patient demise. If liver transplantation is contemplated in a patient with POPH, then the state of the right ventricle must be carefully assessed as any dysfunction of the RV will cause liver graft congestion and possible failure and this may result in the loss of the graft and the patient.

Portopulmonary Hypertension

Portopulmonary hypertension is defined as pulmonary hypertension associated with portal hypertension. The diagnostic criteria for POPH include a mean pulmonary artery pressure (mPAP) of greater than 25 mmHg at rest together with a PVR greater than 240 dynes.s.cm^{-5} and a transpulmonary gradient of greater than 12 mmHg. [2] The pulmonary artery inclusion pressure (PAOP) of less than 15 mmHg is usually included in the definition but in many of the patients with end-stage liver disease there is a very hyperdynamic circulation, volume overload and in some patients a significant cirrhotic cardiomyopathy. These complications may cause an elevation in the pulmonary artery occlusion pressure in addition to the patient having an elevated PVR. Therefore the PAOP of less than 15 mm Hg may exclude patients with true POPH that have these confounding factors. The transpulmonary gradient (mPAP-PAOP) is a measure of the obstruction to blood flow across the pulmonary circulation and distinguishes the contribution of volume from PVR to the increases in mPAP [3]. This is important as approximately 20% of patients with end-stage liver disease presenting for liver transplantation will have elevated pulmonary artery pressures but this is the result of pulmonary venous hypertension and the PVR is normal or low. True POPH with an elevated PVR occurs in approximately 5-6% of liver transplant patients and is caused by pathological changes in the pulmonary arterioles that increase the resistance to blood flow and the work of the RV. It is a progressive disease with a life expectancy of approximately 2 years without liver transplantation [4]. More recent reports have shown some improvement in these survival numbers and may reflect better vasodilator therapy [5,6]. Portopulmonary hypertension may be ameliorated temporarily by pulmonary vasodilator therapy and this should be used to optimize patients for liver transplantation. Many patients will have their POPH reversed with liver transplantation but in some patients the POPH will continue after liver transplantation and in other patients POPH may develop *de novo* after a successful liver transplant. [7,8]

Pathophysiology

The etiology of POPH has not been clearly defined but the histological changes are very similar to those changes found in primary pulmonary hypertension. The pulmonary arteriole vascular wall may exhibit medial hypertrophy, plexiform lesions, intimal proliferation and adventitial fibrosis. It is possible that in the group of patients that fail to respond to liver transplantation some of the patients may have true primary pulmonary hypertension and not POPH. The condition is progressive and when it reaches the fibrosis stage it is very unlikely that it can be repaired and perhaps if this stage could be identified a combined double-lung liver transplant may be considered.

The increased blood flow in the pulmonary arterioles is associated with the typical high cardiac output state that occurs with portal hypertension and liver cirrhosis. This creates stress sheer forces on the vascular endothelium and may well be the cause of endothelial dysfunction [9,10]. The vascular endothelium is the modulator of hemodynamics and as it becomes dysfunctional it can no longer maintain this role. Increased levels of endothelin-1, a potent vasoconstrictor produced by the endothelium are found in POPH, and also reports of increased levels of other vasoactive molecules and inflammatory molecules such as angiotensin 1, thromboxane B2, and prostaglandin $F_2\alpha$. [11, 12] Vasodilator substances such as nitric oxide and prostacyclin synthase may be reduced or in some areas of the pulmonary circulation produced in excess. The result of this is that sometimes hepatopulmonary syndrome (HPS) may be found, caused by the vascular dilatations producing effective pulmonary shunts. HPS may co-exist with POPH in the same patient, with one or the other pathological states predominating [13]. On top of theses pathological changes, the dysfunctional endothelium may not produce adequate thrombomodulin and microthrombosis may occur causing an acute increase in PVR, mPAP and acute RV dysfunction [14]. In the early stages the vasoconstriction is reversible with pulmonary vasodilator therapy. There have also been some genetic links to the cause of pulmonary hypertension and biomarkers have been sought by investigators for the etiology of POPH. Mutation in the gene that codes bone morphogenic protein receptor type 11 has been associated with primary pulmonary hypertension but has not yet been identified in patients with POPH. Other possible risk factors for developing POPH have been identified as the female sex and autoimmune hepatitis [12]. Other studies have implicated genetic variation in estrogen signaling and cell growth regulators as being potential risk factors[15 - 17].

Presentation

The clinical presentation of POPH maybe masked by the symptoms of the underlying liver disease and portal hypertension. Dyspnea on exertion, fatigue, weakness and orthopnea are frequently seen. Moderate hypoxemia and a decreased arterial partial pressure of carbon dioxide have been reported [18]. The electrocardiogram may show a right heart strain pattern including a right bundle branch block. Serum B-type natriuretic peptide may be found to be elevated [19].

If patients are not screened for POPH at initial assessment for liver transplantation, it may not be discovered until the time of transplantation. At this time a careful evaluation made under the pressure of a donor graft being present on ice, must be made. The correct decision on whether to go forward with liver transplantation is crucial as both the graft and the patient's outcome are at risk.

Screening

Every patient presenting with for liver transplantation, with portal hypertension should be screened by two-dimensional Doppler transthoracic echocardiography (TEE) to detect possible pulmonary hypertension [20-23]. The TEE allows the estimation of right ventricular systolic pressure (RVSP) provided there is a tricuspid regurgitant jet present. The RVSP is calculated from the peak tricuspid regurgitant jet velocity (TRV) using the modified Bernoulli equation and estimating the right atrial pressure (RAP): RVSP = $4(TRV)^2$ + RAP. This evaluation, if it can be made has a 97% sensitivity and 77% specificity for diagnosing moderate and severe POPH. [22] If the RSVP is found to be greater than 50 mm Hg a right heart catheterization is indicated to fully characterize the hemodynamic data. Recently a potentially more accurate screening test has been reported utilizing the ratio of peak TVR to the right ventricular outflow tract velocity time integral. This value provides an accurate test for identifying a PVR of more than 120 dyne.s.cm^{-5} [23]. The sensitivity and negative predictive value of this test was reported as 100%. It is also vital that both right and left ventricular anatomy and function are well characterized, taking in to account that the typical patient with cirrhosis has an elevated cardiac output and low systemic vascular resistance. This may give the impression of a dynamic functioning heart and mask significant cirrhotic cardiomyopathy that has been reported to occur in 100% of patients with liver cirrhosis [24]. Any dilation of the right heart chambers must be noted as the risk to undergoing liver transplantation is right heart dysfunction or failure with graft congestion and subsequent graft loss and potential loss of the recipient. The RV in the presence of reduced contractility is very sensitive to increases in workload and will become dysfunctional and fail [25].

Most patients that have pulmonary hypertension presenting for liver transplantation do not have true POPH. On close examination of the pulmonary hemodynamics, most of these patients will have a normal or low PVR and are suffering from volume overload, high output failure or cardiomyopathy with ventricular dysfunction, or a combination of all of these factors. True POPH is only found in 5-6% of transplant candidates and is the result of pathological changes in the pulmonary vasculature. [4]. However true POPH can also exist complicated by volume overload, high output failure and cardiomyopathy, so guidelines on management must be tempered by these possible confounding pathologies. It is also the reason that a normal PAOP does not always fit in the definition of POPH. An elevated PAOP is very compatible and is frequently seen with true POPH. The critical factors are the elevated TPG > 12 mm HG and a PVR > 240 dyne.s.cm^{-5} which have to be determined by right heart catheterization.

If pulmonary hypertension is identified some centers perform a vasodilator challenge to test the potential pulmonary vascular reactivity to give an indication of possible reversibility. This may help with the decision to transplant or not as after liver transplantation the POPH may resolve if it will reverse with drug therapy. If an acute rise in POPH occurs in the perioperative period this may also give a strategy on how to treat it. Possibly vasoreactivity gives an indication that a fixed pathology such as fibrosis in the pulmonary arterioles has not occurred giving hope that a liver transplant may reverse the pathology. However this hypothesis has not yet been tested with a randomized controlled clinical trial. In one vasoreactivity trial, inhaled nitric oxide has been compared to intravenous epoprostenol and oral isosorbide-5-mononitrate in patients with POPH and the results have demonstrated variable reductions in pulmonary hemodynamics [26]

Pharmacotherapy

Once diagnosed with POPH the patient should be treated to optimize the PVR and RV function for potential liver transplantation. Unlike HPS that is reversed by liver transplantation POPH may not reverse immediately and may require prolonged vasodilator therapy. In a few patients undergoing liver transplantation the POPH will not reverse and these patients cannot be predicted ahead of time.

The institution of diuretic therapy can reduce the hypervolemia that may be a significant component of the presentation of an elevated mPAP, and can certainly reduce the CVP and chamber dilatation.

The use of calcium channel blockers are contraindicated in the treatment of POPH as they have been demonstrated to increase the hepatic venous gradient and portal vein flow in cirrhotic patients [27]. Beta-blockers have also been demonstrated to adversely affect hemodynamics [28].

Epoprostenol an analogue of prostaglandin I_2 is a potent pulmonary arteriole vasodilator. It is an intravenous agent that because of its short half-life requires a continuous infusion via an indwelling catheter. This poses a potential infection risk over the long term that it frequently needed. Epoprostenol is also an inhibitor of platelet function; causes splenomegaly and these both may have a significant negative impact on the effect of the existing thrombocytopenia usually found in th cirrhotic patient [29]. Other side effects associated with long-term intravenous epoprostenol include jaw pain, headache, flushing, nausea and other unpleasant symptoms. However therapy with epoprostenol has been shown to be effective in some patients by improving the pulmonary hemodynamics and allowing time for RV function to improve, mPAP to ameliorate and allow successful liver transplantation[30-32]. Sudden cessation of the epoprostenol infusion may result in rebound vasoconstriction, severe pulmonary hypertension and potential death and so must be avoided.

Other prostacyclin analogues have been trialed in clinical case series with some positive outcomes. Iloprost may be administered intravenously but has the advantage that it can be delivered via an inhaler. The length of action is short and requires frequent administration, up to 6 to 9 times a day but it does avoid the need for an indwelling catheter [33, 34]. In an experimental animal model inhaled iloprost was shown to improve global hemodynamics [35]. Intravenous iloprost has been used as a bridge to liver transplantation in patients with POPH [36].

Treprostinil has been administered over the long term subcutaneously with some positive results [37]; treprostinil also may be administered intravenously.

Endothelin receptor antagonists block the vasoconstrictive action of endothelin-1 on the pulmonary vasculature. They have the advantage that they may be given orally. Bosentan is a dual endothelin receptor antagonist blocking both endothelin A and B receptors so that endothelin-1 cannot bind and cause vasoconstriction. Bosentan has been associated with an increase in hepatic enzymes in a small percentage of patients on initiation of therapy [38,39].

However, in a group of patients with severe POPH bosentan and iloprost were shown to be safe and the bosentan group had better long-term survival [34]. Ambrisentan is another endothelin-1 receptor blocker that has just been approved for the treatment of primary pulmonary hypertension with no reported hepatic adverse effects and this may be a more suitable agent for treating POPH [40].

The phosphodiesterase 5 inhibitor, sildenafil is another oral drug that has shown efficacy in treating POPH. [41,42] The cyclic guanosine monophosphatase-specific phosphodiesterase type 5 enzymes that are found in the pulmonary vascular endothelium are selectively inhibited. This prolongs the effects of nitric oxide (NO) mediated vasodilatation in the endothelium [43].

Inhaled milrinone, a phosphodiesterase-3 inhibitor, has been used as a selective pulmonary vasodilator, when delivered via a nebulizer system, in cardiac surgery and may have a role in the treatment of decompensated pulmonary hypertension in liver transplantation. When administered as an inhalant milrinone does not cause systemic hypotension [44].

Chronic inhalation of NO has been used in the treatment of primary pulmonary hypertension and also to reverse acute elevations in mPAP during liver transplantation. [45,46}

Combination therapies of these drugs have been used with some success [47].

New antiproliferative therapies that block the platelet-derived growth factor receptor may allow a reversal of the vascular remodeling and cause a reduction in POPH are under review [48].

Staging of POPH: Risk Management

The risk of undergoing liver transplantation in the patient with POPH has been assessed based on the mPAP and an experience based on case reports, case series, local databases and a small national database. However mixed pathologies may exist in this patient group including volume overload, high cardiac output and cirrhotic cardiomyopathy that will alter the risks of going ahead with transplantation. The key factors to survival rest with the RV function and the level of fixed resistance to the outflow of the RV, which is a function of the PVR more than the actual value of them PAP. However it is a good starting point to trigger a risk evaluation.

A patient who has compensated well to an increase in PVR by a strengthening of the RV may successfully undergo a liver transplant with a high mPAP than a patient who has poorly compensated and has a low mPAP.

As a guide, in patients with an elevated PVR, an mPAP of 25 mmHg to 35 mm Hg is termed mild POPH and does not have an increased risk for transplantation. Moderate POPH is an mPAP of 35 to 45 mm Hg and this has a significantly increased mortality of up to 50% . Severe POPH, an mPAP of greater than 45 mm Hg has up to 100% mortality. [49] The critical factor in each patient undergoing liver transplantation is whether the RV is able to handle the increases in mPAP caused by increases in volume, and significant increases in cardiac output against a potentially fixed resistance to flow. Therefore in the preoperative assessment the acute response to vasodilator therapy may give good information on how the patient will respond intraoperatively. A challenge with volume and a dobutamine infusion to increase cardiac output while observing RV function by echocardiography may also be helpful in assessing how the patient may tolerate transplantation.

The speed of onset of POPH is not known. However whenever endothelial dysfunction occurs there is the possibility of pulmonary microthrombosis and an acute rise in PVR and mPAP. Patients who are diagnosed with POPH should be started on vasodilator therapy and periodically undergo reassessment for suitability for liver transplantation. The screening for POPH and the aggressive treatment with pulmonary vasodilator therapy to reverse the process and optimize the patient for liver transplantation has improved the outcomes of this patient group [50-54].

POPH Risk Assessment Algorithm:

5. All liver transplant candidates screened by TTE
    If RVSP > than 50 mm Hg perform right heart catheterization
6. 2. mPAP < 35 mm Hg and PVR 250 − 300 dyne.s.cm^{-5}, good RV function: start on vasodilator therapy and place on transplant waiting list. Reassess every 6 months or if clinical deterioration. At time of transplant recheck with right heart catheter and TEE in the operating room prior to starting surgery.
7. mPAP 35 to 45 mm Hg and PVR 250 to 350 dyne.s.cm^{-5}, test reversibility, assess RV function, start on vasodilator therapy. If RV function good, stress with volume and dobutamine. If RV fails test or function is reduced defer surgery and monitor effect of chronic

vasodilator therapy. If RV function excellent consider going ahead with transplant.
8. mPAP > 45 mm Hg and PVR t greater than 250 dyne.s.cm^{-5} treat with vasodilator therapy and defer transplant until mPAP improved and RV function good.
9. Following transplant continue to treat mPAP and PVR until values normalized.

Perioperative Management

If POPH is first diagnosed on the operating table immediately prior to liver transplantation a careful assessment of the pulmonary hemodynamics and RV function must be made with a right heart catheterization and transesophageal echocardiograph (TEE). If mPAP < 35 mm Hg and RV good then consider going ahead with transplant as long as CVP is normal. Otherwise defer transplant until pulmonary hemodynamics and RV can be optimized.

If the patient has known POPH and has been treated then a careful reassessment has to be made to be sure that there has been no deterioration in RV function. As the patient may have had deterioration in renal function with resulting volume overload continuous venovenous hemodialysis may be necessary if the vascular filling pressures are elevated. This can easily be instituted in the operating room at the time of surgery.

The intraoperative management of the patient requires both right heart catheterization and TEE monitoring to manage the perturbations of the procedure. The key strategies to optimal management include reducing PVR and preventing acute rises in PVR and maintain good RV function. Monitor for early signs of RV decompensation so that early interventions can be made before the patient or the new graft become compromised. Systemic perfusion pressure must be maintained to prevent right ventricular ischemia and sinus rhythm should be maintained to allow adequate RV filling. Maintenance of normocapnia, and avoidance of hypoxia with the early treatment of acidosis and hypothermia are essential in preventing a rise in PVR [55]. These considerations also apply postoperatively in the critical care unit and early weaning from mechanical ventilation and extubation should not be considered in this very high acuity group of patients.

Liver Transplantation and Pulmonary Hypertension 127

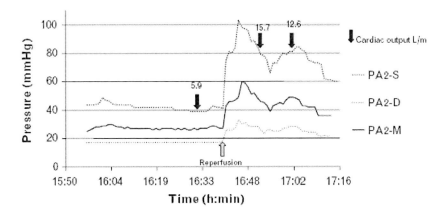

Figure 1 Increase in cardiac output with concomitant increase in pulmonary artery pressures at reperfusion of the liver graft.
PA2-S, pulmonary artery pressure-systolic; PA2-D, pulmonary artery pressure – diastolic; PA2-M, pulmonary artery pressure – mean.
Reprinted with permission from Ramsay M. *Advances in Pulmonary Hypertension 2004;2:9-18.*[2]

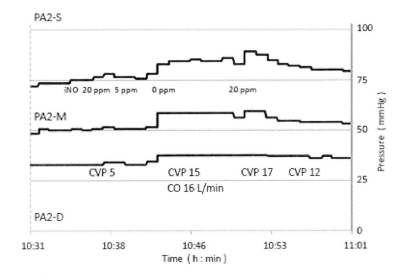

Figure 2. The effect of withdrawing inhaled nitric oxide on right heart function following liver transplantation. Note the rise in CVP from 5 mm Hg to 17 mm Hg and then reducing to 12 mm Hg on restarting the nitric oxide.
PA2-S, pulmonary artery pressure-systolic; PA2-D, pulmonary artery pressure – diastolic; PA2-M, pulmonary artery pressure – mean. CVP, central venous pressure, CO, cardiac output.

Acute Decompensated Pulmonary Hypertension

A strategy must be in place before starting the liver transplant on how to manage an acute decompensation in RV function caused by an elevation in mPAP. The new graft will quickly become congested and fail unless urgent effective therapy is undertaken to rapidly reduce mPAP and PVR. The period of highest risk is at the time of reperfusion of the graft. This is when an increase in cardiac output may occur up to 300% of the baseline value [3]. This massive increase in flow facing a fixed resistance in the pulmonary vasculature may cause a very large and rapid increase in mPAP. Figure 1.

The effect of an ischemia/reperfusion injury on the vascular endothelium may compound the deleterious effects of this critical event [56,57]. Inotropic therapy to assist the RV contractility may be required such as dobutamine or inhaled milrinone. Early initiation of pulmonary vasodilators is essential. Inhaled nitric oxide has been shown to be effective in some instances [46].Figure 2 Inhaled iloprost is another therapy that may be effective but the nebulizer and the administration tools for these agents must be immediately available. Vasopressin may have a role in maintaining systemic pressure as under experimental conditions it produces pulmonary vasodilatation and systemic vasoconstriction, but this has not been confirmed consistently in the clinical environment [58].

Other potential therapies include the use of an intra-aortic balloon pump to maintain left ventricular function, a right ventricular assist device and even a balloon septoplasty to create an ASD to decompress the right heart.

Postoperative Care

These patients can be expected to have a prolonged and critical recovery period. All the intraoperative measures need to be maintained to prevent a rebound of pulmonary hypertension during this period.

The role of liver transplantation in the treatment of POPH is not well defined. There are case reports of complete reversal of POPH after liver transplantation but there are other case series where pulmonary vasodilator has had to be continued for the long term [59-64]. There are other reports of progression of POPH after transplantation and eventual demise of the patient [65]. There may be a window of opportunity for carefully assessed patients who respond to vasodilator therapy to undergo early transplantation. The United Network for Organ Sharing (UNOS) is considering making an exception for those patients diagnosed with POPH and responds effectively to vasodilator therapy [66].

A therapeutic option for the patient with a fixed PVR and moderate to severe POPH maybe a combined lung and liver transplant [67]. The overall survival in one case series of 10 patients who underwent a double lung and liver transplant was at 1, 3and 5 years: 69, 62 and 49% respectively.

Conclusion

The etiology of POPH has not been fully elucidated. The effect of portal hypertension is to cause endothelial dysfunction in the pulmonary arterioles. This may result in a vasodilatation process HPS, or a proliferative process POPH or both entities may exist together. Which patients with portal hypertension will develop POPH is unknown. The key to understanding which patients with POPH will tolerate liver transplantation is the RV function. Impaired RV function will cause graft congestion with possible loss of graft and potential patient demise. Therefore those patients that do not respond to vasodilator therapy with a reduction in PVR and mPAP and with improvement in RV function are a relative contraindication to liver transplantation. Other factors to be considered are the impact of volume overload, high cardiac output and cirrhotic cardiomyopathy. Transplantation has been successful in patients who have responded to vasodilator therapy and many patients have been able to be weaned off therapy in the months post transplantation. However there are reports that even a successful liver transplant in this patient group does not guarantee a reversal of the pathological process. Careful assessment and optimization of the patient with POPH is necessary to delineate the risks of undergoing liver transplantation and whether this is the right therapy for the patient.

References

[1] Mantz FA, Craig E. Portal axis thrombosis with spontaneous portacaval shunt and resultant cor pulmonale. *Arch Pathol Lab Med* 1951; 52:91-97

[2] Rodriguez-Roisin R, Krowka M, Hervé P, Fallon M. ERS Task Force Pulmonary-Hepatic Vascular Disorders (PHD) Scientific Committee. Pulmonary-Hepatic Vascular Disorders. *Eur Respir J* 2004; 24:861-880.

[3] Ramsay M. Portopulmonary hypertension and right heart failure in patients with Cirrhosis. *Curr Opin Anaesthesiol* 2010; 23:145-150.
[4] Herve P, Lebrec D, Brenot F, Simonneau G, Humbert M, Sitbon O, Duroux P. Pulmonary vascular disorders in portal hypertension. *Eur Resp J* 1998; 11:1153-66.
[5] Kawut SM, Krowka MJ, Trotter JF, Roberts KE, Benza RL, Badesch DB, Taichman DB, Horn EM, Zacks S, Kaplowitz N, Brown RS Jr, Fallon MB; Pulmonary Vascular Complications of Liver Disease Study Group.Clinical risk factors for portopulmonary hypertension. *Hepatology* 2008; 48:196-203.
[6] Le Pavec J, Souza R, Herve P, Lebrec D, Savale L, Tcherakian C, Jaïs X, Yaïci A, Humbert M, Simonneau G, Sitbon O. Portopulmonary hypertension: Survival and prognostic factors. *Am J Respir Crit Care Med* 2008; 178:637-643.
[7] Koch DG, Caplan M, Reuben A. Pulmonary hypertension after liver transplantation: Case presentation and review of the literature. *Liver Transpl* 2009; 15:407-412.
[8] Ramsay M. Liver transplantation and pulmonary hypertension: pathophysiology and management strategies. *Curr Opin Organ Transplant* 2007; 12:274-280.
[9] Schroeder RA, Ewing CA, Sitzmann JV, Kuo PC. Pulmonary expression of iNOS and HO-1 protein is upregulated in a rat model of prehepatic portal hypertension. *Dig Dis Sci.* 2000;4 5(12):2405-10
[10] Ramsay M. Portopulmonary hypertension and hepatopulmonary syndrome and liver transplantation. *Int Anesthesiol Clin* 2006; 44:69-82.
[11] Bernardi M, Gulberg V, Colantoni A, Trevisani F, Gasbarrini A, Gerbes AL. Plasma endothelin-1 and 3 in cirrhosis: relationship with systemic hemodynamics, renal function and neurohumeral systems. *J Hepatol* 1996, 24: 161-168.
[12] Maruyama T, Ohsaki K, Shimoda S, Kaji Y, Harada M. Thromboxane-dependent portopulmonary hypertension. *Am J Med* 2005; 118; 93-94.
[13] Kaspar MD, Ramsay MA, Shuey CB Jr, Levy MF, Klintmalm GG. Severe pulmonary hypertension and amelioration of hepatopulmonary syndrome after liver transplantation. *Liver Transpl Surg.* 1998 Mar;4(2):177-9
[14] Newman JH. Pulmonary hypertension *Am J Respir Crit Care Med.* 2005; 172(9):1072-7
[15] Roberts KE, Fallon MB, Krowka MD, Brown RS, Trotter JF, Peter I, Tighiouart H, Knowles JA, Rabinowitz D, Benza RL, Badesch DB,

Taichman DB, Horn EM, Zacks S, Kaplowitz N, Kawut SM; Pulmonary Vascular Complications of Liver Disease Study Group*et.* Genetic risk factors for portopulmonary hypertension in patients with advanced liver disease. *Am J Respir Crit Care Med* 2009; 179:835-842.

[16] Roberts KE, Fallon MB, Krowka MJ, Benza RL, Knowles JA, Badesch DB, Brown RS Jr, Taichman DB, Trotter J, Zacks S, Horn EM, Kawut SM; Pulmonary Vascular Complications of Liver Disease Study Group Serotonin transporter polymorphisms in patients with portopulmonary hypertension. *Chest* 2009; 135:1470-1475.

[17] Peng T, Zamanian R, Krowka MJ, Benza RL, Roberts KE, Taichman DB, Rybak D, Trotter JF, Brown RS Jr, Fallon MB, Kawut SM; Pulmonary Vascular Complications of Liver Disease Study Group. *Biomarkers.* 2009 May;14(3):156-60.

[18] Swanson KL, Krowka MJ. Arterial oxygenation associated with portopulmonary hypertension. *Chest.* 2002;121(6):1869-75

[19] Bernal V, Pascual I, Esquivias P, García-Gil A, Mateo JM, Lacambra I, Serrano MT, Simón MA. N-Terminal brain natriuretic peptide as a diagnostic test in cirrhotic patients with pulmonary arterial hypertension. *Transplant Proc* 2009; 41:987-988.

[20] Colle IO, Moreau R, Godinho E, Belghiti J, Ettori F, Cohen-Solal A, Mal H, Bernuau J, Marty J, Lebrec D, Valla D, Durand F. Diagnosis of portopulmonary hypertension in candidates for liver transplantation. *Hepatology* 2003; 37: 401-409.

[21] Murray KF, Carithers RL Jr. AASLD practice guidelines: evaluation of the patient for liver transplantation. *Hepatology* 2005; 41: 1407-1432.

[22] Kim W, Krowka M, Plevak D, Lee J, Rettke SR, Frantz RP, Wiesner RHAccuracy of Doppler echocardiography in the assessment of pulmonary hypertension in liver transplant candidates. *Liver Transpl* 2000; 6:453-458.

[23] Farzaneh-Far R, McKeown BH, Dang D, Roberts J, Schiller NB, Foster E Accuracy of Doppler-estimated pulmonary vascular resistance in patients before liver transplantation. *Am J Cardiol* 2008; 101:259-262.

[24] Alqahtani SA, Fouad TR, Lee SS. Cirrhotic cardiomyopathy. *Semin Liver Dis.* 2008;28(1):59-69. Review.

[25] Afifi S, Shayan S, Al-Qamari A. Pulmonary hypertension and right ventricular function: interdependence in pathophysiology and management. *Int Anesthesiol Clin* 2009;47:97-120

[26] Ricci GL, Melgosa MT, Burgos F, Valera JL, Pizarro S, Roca J, Rodriquez-Roisin R, Barbara JA. Assessment of acute pulmonary vascular reactivity in portopulmonary hypertension. *Liver Transpl* 2007; 13:1506-1514.

[27] Ota K, Shijo H, Kokawa H, Kubara K, Kim T, Akiyoshi N, Yokoyama M, Okumura M. Effects of nifedipine on hepatic venous pressure gradient and portal vein blood flow in patients with cirrhosis. *J Gastroenterol Hepatol* 1995; 10: 198-204.

[28] Provencher S, Herve P, Jais X, Lebrec D, Humbert M, Simonneau G, Sitbon O. Deleterious effects of beta-blockers on exercise capacity and hemodynamics in patients with portopulmonary hypertension. *Gastroenterology.* 2006;130(1):120-126.

[29] Findlay JY, Plevak DJ, Krowka MJ, Sack EM, Porayko MK. Progressive splenomegaly after epoprostenol therapy in portopulmonary hypertension. *Liver Transpl Surg* 1999; 5: 362-365.

[30] Fix OK, Bass NM, De Marco T, Merriman RB. Long-term follow-up of portopulmonary hypertension: effect of treatment with epoprostenol. *Liver Transpl* 2007; 13: 875-885.

[31] Krowka MJ, Frantz RP, McGoon MD, Severson C, Plevak DJ, Weisner RH. Improvement in pulmonary hemodynamics during intravenous epoprostenol (prostacyclin): a study of 15 patients with moderate to severe portopulmonary hypertension. *Hepatology* 1999; 30: 641-648.

[32] Kuo PC, Johnson LB, Plotkin JS, Howell CD, Bartlett ST, Rubin LJ. Continuous intravenous infusion of epoprostenol for the treatment of portopulmonary hypertension. *Transplantation* 1997; 63: 604-606.

[33] Krug S, Sablotzki A, Hammerschmidt S, Wirtz H, Seyfarth HJ. Inhaled iloprost for the control of pulmonary hypertension. *Vasc Health and Risk Mgmt,* 2009:5:465-474.

[34] Hoeper M, Seyfarth H, Hoeffken G, Wirtz H, Spiekerkoetter E, Pletz MW, Welte T, Halank M. Experience with inhaled iloprost and bosentan in portopulmonary hypertension. *Eur Respir J* 2007; 30: 1096-1102.

[35] Rex S, Missant C, Claus P, Buhre W, Wouters PF. Effects of inhaled iloprost on right ventricular contractility, right ventriculo-vascular coupling and ventricular interdependence: a randomized placebo-controlled trial in an experimental model of acute pulmonary hypertension. *Crit Care* 2008, 12: 1-13.

[36] Minder S, Fischler M, Muelhaupt B, Zalunardo MP, Jenni R, Clavien PA, Speich R. Intravenous iloprost bridging to orthotopic liver transplantation in portopulmonary hypertension. *Eur Respir J* 2004; 24: 703-707.

[37] Benza RL, Rayburn BK, Tallaj JA, Pamboukian SV, Bourge RC. Treprostinil-based therapy in the treatment of moderate-to-severe pulmonary arterial hypertension: long-term efficacy and combination with bosentan. *Chest.* 2008 Jul;134(1):139-45
[38] Rubin LJ, Badesch DB, Barst RJ, Galie N, Black CM, Keogh A, Pulido T, Frost A, Roux S, Leconte I, Landzberg M, Simonneau G. Bosentan therapy for pulmonary artery hypertension . *N Engl J Med* 2002; 346: 896-903.
[39] Galiè N, Rubin Lj, Hoeper M, Jansa P, Al-Hiti H, Meyer G, Chiossi E, Kusic-Pajic A, Simonneau G. Treatment of patients with mildly symptomatic pulmonary arterial hypertension with bosentan (EARLY study): a double-blind, randomised controlled trial. *Lancet.* 2008 Jun 21;371(9630):2093-100
[40] McGoon MD, Frost AE, Oudiz RJ, Badesch DB, Galie N, Olschewski H, McLaughlin VV, Gerber MJ, Dufton C, Despain DJ, Rubin LJ. Ambrisentan therapy in patients with pulmonary arterial hypertension who discontinued bosentan or sitaxsentan due to liver function test abnormalities. *Chest.* 2009 Jan;135(1):122-9.
[41] Gough M, White J. Sildenafil therapy is associated with improved hemodynamics in liver transplantation candidates with pulmonary artery hypertension. *Liver Transpl* 2009; 15: 30-36.
[42] Hemnes A, Robbins I. Sildenafil monotherapy in portopulmonary hypertension can facilitate liver transplantation. *Liver Transpl* 2009; 15: 15-19.
[43] Montani D, Chaumais MC, Savale L, Natali D, Price LC, Jaïs X, Humbert M, Simonneau G, Sitbon O. Phosphodiesterase type 5 inhibitors in pulmonary arterial hypertension. *Adv Ther.* 2009;26(9):813-25.
[44] Wang H, Gong M, Bin Z, Dai A. Comparison of inhaled and intravenous milrinone in patients with pulmonary hypertension undergoing mitral valve surgery. *Adv Ther* 2009; 26:462-468.
[45] Findlay JY, Harrison BA, Plevak DJ, Krowka MJ. Inhaled nitric oxide reduces pulmonary artery pressures in portopulmonary hypertension. *Liver Transpl Surg.* 1999;5(5):381-7
[46] Ramsay MAE, Spikes C, East CA, et al. The perioperative management of portopulmonary hypertension with nitric oxide and epoprostenol. *Anesthesiology* 1999; 90:299-301.
[47] Austin MJ, McDougall NI, Wendon JA, Sizer E, Knisely AS, Rela M, Wilson C, Callender ME, O'Grady JG, Heneghan MA. Safety and efficacy of combined use of sildenafil, bosentan, and iloprost before and after liver

transplantation in severe portopulmonary hypertension. *Liver Transpl.* 2008;14(3):287-91.

[48] Tapper E, Knowles D, Heffron T, Lawrence EC, Csete M. Portopulmonary hypertension: imatinib as a novel treatment and the Emory experience with this condition. *Transpl Proc* 2009; 1:1969-1971.

[49] Swanson KL, Wiesner RH, Nyberg SL, Rosen CB, Krowka MJ. Survival in portopulmonary hypertension: Mayo Clinic experience categorized by treatment subgroups. *Am J Transplant* 2008; 8:2445-2453.

[50] Swanson KL, Krowka MJ. Screen for portopulmonary hypertension, especially in liver transplant candidates. *Cleve Clin J Med* 2008; 75:121-136.

[51] Ashfaq M, Chinnakotla S, Rodgers L.Ausloos K, Saadeh S, Klintmalm GB, Ramsay M, Davis GL. The impact of treatment of portopulmonary *hypertension on survival following liver transplantation.* Am J Transpl 2007; 7:1258-1264.

[52] Krowka M, Mandell M, Ramsay M, Kawut SM, Fallon MB, Manzarbeitia C, Pardo M Jr, Marotta P, Uemoto S, Stoffel MP, Benson JT Hepatopulmonary syndrome and portopulmonary hypertension: a report of the multicenter liver transplant database. *Liver Transpl* 2004; 10:174-182.

[53] Naeije R, Huez S. Expert opinion on available options treating pulmonary arterial hypertension. *Expert Opin Pharmacother* 2007; 8: 2247-2265.

[54] Porres-Aguilar M, ZuckermanM, Figueroa-Casas J, Krowka M. Portopulmonary hypertension: state of the art. *Ann Hepatol* 2008; 7: 321-330.

[55] Zamanian RT, Haddad F, Doyle RL, Weinacker A. Management strategies for patients with pulmonary hypertension in the intensive care unit. *Crit Care Med.* 2007;35(9):2037-50. Review

[56] Ramsay M. The reperfusion syndrome: have we made any progress? *Liver Transpl.* 2008 Apr;14(4):412-4.

[57] Paugam-Burtz C, Kavafyan J, Merckx P, Dahmani S, Sommacale D, Ramsay M, Belghiti J, Mantz J. Postreperfusion syndrome during liver transplantation for cirrhosis: outcome and predictors. *Liver Transpl.* 2009; 15(5):522-9

[58] Braun EB, Palin CA, Hogue CW. Vasopressin during spinal anesthesia in a patient with primary pulmonary hypertension treated with intravenous epoprostenol. *Anesth Analg* 2004; 99: 36-37.

[59] Sugimachi K, Soejima Y, Morita S, Ueda S, Fukuhara T, Nagata S, Ikegami T, Taketomi A, Maehara Y. Rapid normalization of portopulmonary

hypertension after living donor liver transplantation. *Transpl Proc* 2009; 41: 1976-1978.
[60] Umeda N, Kamath P. Hepatopulmonary syndrome and portopulmonary hypertension. *Hepatol Res* 2009; 39: 1020-1022.
[61] Swanson K, Wiesner R, Nyberg S. Rosen CB, Krowka MJ. Survival in portopulmonary hypertension: Mayo Clinic experience categorized by treatment subgroups. *Am J Transpl* 2008; 8: 2445-2453.
[62] Singh C, Sager J. Pulmonary complications of cirrhosis. *Med Clin N Am.* 2009; 95: 871-883.
[63] Yeshua H, Blendis L, Oren R. Pulmonary manifestations of liver diseases *Sem Cardiothorac Vasc Anesth* 2009; 13: 60-69.
[64] Golbin J, Krowka M. Portopulmonary hypertension. *Clin Chest Med* 2007; 28: 203-218.
[65] Krowka MJ, Mandell MS, Ramsay MA, Kawut SM, Fallon MB, Manzarbeitia C, Pardo M Jr, Marotta P, Uemoto S, Stoffel MP, Benson JT. Hepatopulmonary syndrome and portopulmonary hypertension: a report of the multicenter liver transplant database. *Liver Transpl.* 2004;10(2):174-82.
[66] Krowka M, Fallon M, Mulligan D et al. Model for end-stage liver disease (MELD) exception for portopulmonary hypertension. *Liver Transpl* 2006; 12: S114-S116.
[67] Grannas G, NeippM, Hoeper M, et al. Indications for and outcomes after combined lung and liver transplantation: a single center experience on 13 consecutive cases. *Transplantation* 2008; 85: 524-531.

In: Pulmonary Hypertension
Editor: Huili Gan

ISBN: 978-1-61470-556-7
© 2012 Nova Science Publishers, Inc.

Chapter VI

Pulmonary Hypertension in the Down Syndrome Population

Clifford L. Cua[*,a], *Louis G. Chicoine*[b], *Leif D. Nelin*[b], *and Mary Mullen*[c]

[a] Heart Center, [b]Section of Neonatology, Department of Pediatrics, [a, b] Nationwide Children's Hospital and the Department of Cardiology, [c]Children's Hospital Boston

Abstract

Down syndrome (DS) is a common genetic disorder with protean manifestations. Children with DS are at risk for multiple medical issues that are well described; however, a potentially underappreciated condition that appears to have a high prevalence in this patient population is pulmonary hypertension (PH). The increased prevalence of PH in this population may have serious short and long-term consequences. The causes of PH in the DS population are not precisely known, but may be due to multiple other associated medical conditions that these children have concurrently, or due to shared biological features. We review the literature that describes the possible

---

[*] Corresponding author, Assistant Professor of Pediatrics, Heart Center, Department of Pediatrics, Nationwide Children's Hospital. 700 Children's Drive, Columbus, OH 43205, Bus: 614-722-2530, Fax: 614-722-2549, Email: clcua@hotmail.com

etiologies of PH in DS children with the hope that further research is performed to better define this complicated population.

Keywords: Down syndrome, pulmonary hypertension

Introduction

Down syndrome (DS) is a common genetic disorder and the most viable trisomy [1]. Multiple medical problems including neurologic [2], orthopedic [3], endocrinologic [4,5], cardiac [6], gastrointestinal [7,8], oncologic [9,10], and immunologic [11,12] have been associated with this syndrome. One medical condition that has also been associated with DS, but may be underappreciated, is pulmonary hypertension (PH). PH may have serious detrimental consequences in these individuals and should be recognized and treated as soon as diagnosed to improve short and long-term outcomes. Neither the contributors to PH in DS patients, nor the precise incidence or prevalence over time are well established. This review will describe some of the possibilities that may place DS patients at risk for PH.

Several of the medical issues associated with DS may contribute to the development of PH, such as cardiac lesions and respiratory problems. There may also be specific intrinsic biological links between DS and PH that account for the severity in this population. The etiology for PH in DS is almost certainly multi-factorial and may be classified according to the recent WHO/Evian classification for PH [13]. This classification scheme identifies etiologies to PH as associated with disorders of the respiratory system or hypoxemia: 3.1: chronic obstructive pulmonary disease, 3.3: sleep disordered breathing, 3.4: alveolar hypoventilation, 3.6: neonatal lung disease, 3.7: alveolar capillary dysplasia; PH related to 1.2(b): congenital systemic-to-pulmonary shunts, or PH that is 1.1(a) sporadic.

Anatomical upper airway obstruction (UAO) is common in DS. Well described abnormalities that contribute to UAO include macroglossia, tonsillar and adenoidal enlargement, subglottic stenosis, laryngomalacia, and trachea-malacia [14]. These abnormalities may contribute to chronic hypo-ventilation and hypoxemia and thus put the DS patient at risk factor for developing PH [15]. In one study, 53 pediatric (7.4 + 1.2 years) DS patients had nap polysomnograms performed and 77% of the patients studied subsequently had abnormal findings. Findings included obstructive and central apnea, hypoventilation, and oxygen saturations less than 90%. Sixteen of these DS patients additionally had overnight sleep polysomnograms and 100% of them had abnormal findings. Age, obesity, or presence of congenital heart disease (CHD) did not predict abnormal polysomnography studies. The polysomnograms improved in the patients that subsequently underwent tonsillectomy and adenoidectomy, but did not totally normalize in any of the patients [16]. A smaller study with seven DS patients also showed improvement in their polymsomnograms and clinical symptoms after UAO surgery [17]. These observations are consistent with multiple case reports and case series of PH in DS with UAO that either improved or normalized after the obstruction was relieved with removal of the tissue or with placement of a tracheostomy [18-25]. One group reported on a large cohort of patients with UAO and found that premature infants or DS patients with CHD had the highest risk for developing PAH [26]. They also reported on 71 DS patients with UAO, 34 of which had PH, who underwent surgical palliation for UAO. Symptoms and PH frequently improved after surgery, but similar to other studies, did not completely normalize. Nonetheless, 39% still had significant residual symptoms and there were five deaths [27].

In addition to UAO, DS can be associated with abnormalities in the lung parenchyma or vasculature that may predispose to PH, though the data are conflicting. One of the earliest studies examined lung specimens in 82 DS patients. These specimens were matched for age, sex, and CHD in non-DS patients. This study found no significant differences in the pulmonary vasculature from lung specimens from DS versus non-DS patients [28]. However, recent studies have shown abnormalities in DS versus non-DS patients in lung architecture. Lung hypoplasia with decreased number of alveoli in relation to acini as well as enlarged alveolar ducts have been reported in DS versus non-DS patients with lung biopsies [29]. Other investigators have noted differences in the number of type II alveolar cells between DS versus non-DS patients [30]. Case reports have identified alveolar capillary dysplasia in DS patients that lead to intractable PH [31,32], though the low incidence of such dysplasia, in general, makes comparisons between DS and non-DS populations challenging [33]. Collectively, these recent findings point toward substantial differences in lung parenchymal and vasculature changes that may be risk factors for DS patients developing PH.

Another common medical issue in DS is the presence of CHD. DS patients have approximately a 50% incidence of CHD with atrioventricular septal defects (AVSD) and ventricular septal defects (VSD) comprising the vast majority of lesions [6,34]. These lesions allow left-to-right intra-cardiac blood flow resulting in increased pulmonary blood flow, which over time damages the pulmonary vasculature and leads to PH [35]. A specific anatomical lesion seen with AVSD has also been implicated in increasing the risk for PH [36]. Regardless of the mechanism, there is no question that unrepaired CHD associated with a left-to-right shunt is a substantial risk factor for the development of PH [37,38].

While CHD increases the risk of PH, DS patients appear to have a higher incidence of developing PH compared to non-DS patients with CHD [34,37,39-41]. DS patients also appear to have a more significant degree of pre-operative PH compared to non-DS patients with similar CHD lesions. DS has been associated with significantly lower pulmonary blood flow and higher pulmonary vasculature resistance compared to non-DS patients before cardiac surgery and to a higher risk of developing fixed PH at less than one year of age compared to non-DS patients [42]. Moreover, pathological lung specimens have increased pulmonary vasculature intimal changes, pulmonary arterial lumen narrowing, thinning of the arterial media, and fibrotic intimal proliferation in DS patients versus non-DS patients with similar CHD lesions [43,44]. Surgical repair of CHD achieves improvement in pulmonary artery pressures [45-47], but DS patients still appear to have a higher incidence and less resolution of PH post-repair. In a study with 1349 patients less than 18 years of age, the incidence of PH episodes was 9.9% in DS patients versus 1.2% in non-DS patients [48]. An additional study documented a larger decrease in pulmonary vasculature resistance in non-DS patients than in DS patients after VSD repair [49].

Even accounting for multiple risk factors that predispose to developing PH such as UAO or CHD, DS patients also appear to have an increased incidence with greater severity of PH compared to non-DS patients. This observation has led to speculation that DS may directly contribute the risk for PH irrespective of related cardiopulmonary conditions. Examples of this include the demonstration of an increased risk of persistent pulmonary hypertension of the newborn (PPHN) compared non-DS patients regardless of baseline demographics [50]. Another study examined the ELSO database which contained 15,946 patients placed on extracorporeal membrane oxygenation (ECMO) in the neonatal period, of which 91 had DS. This study found that the primary reason for ECMO support was significantly different for DS patients versus non-DS patients with PPHN being the primary reason in 47.3% of the DS patients and only 13% in the non-DS patients. The DS patients also had a greater risk for being placed on ECMO with worse survival than did patients without DS [51]. Both studies suggest that the transition from intra- to extra-uterine life in DS patients may not be normal in regards to the pulmonary vasculature.

Catheterization data suggests that DS patients do not exhibit the same level of pulmonary vasodilatation to nitric oxide (NO) or oxygen as do non-DS patients [52,53]. In the systemic circulation, DS can also be associated with decreased brachial blood flow and a decreased vascular resistance response to acetylcholine administration versus non-DS patients, though the response to nitroglycerin was similar between the two groups of patients. This study implied that NO production is impaired in the DS patient since acetylcholine vasodilation is mediated by NO production in the endothelium whereas nitroglycerin is a direct NO donor [54]. In addition to these differences in physiology, cellular differences may also exist in the lung vasculature. Endothelial progenitor cells, which are central to the maintenance of vascular homeostasis, were shown to be lowest in DS patients with Eisenmenger physiology (i.e. PH associated with CHD) versus non-DS patients with Eisenmenger physiology, idiopathic PH, or controls without PH [55]. Levels of endothelin, a potent endogenously produced vasoconstrictor, were shown to be significantly elevated in DS patients versus non-DS patients pre- and post-CHD surgery. There was a direct correlation between endothelin levels and pulmonary artery pressures [56]. Finally, there have been differences noted in alkaline phosphatase activity, which has a role in pulmonary surfactant secretion, between lung tissue of DS versus non-DS patients [30]. These diverse findings suggest that simply having the diagnosis of DS increases the risk and severity of PH compared to the non-DS population. Genetic variations that predispose to PH have been studied in DS patients, but at this time, there has been no definitive genetic variations identified in DS patients that predispose them to PH [57,58].

There is a growing recognition of the problem of PH in DS patients. Factors important to causing PH in DS include well known congenital abnormalities, but also may reflect intrinsic differences between DS and non-DS individuals. These preliminary clinical and laboratory observations warrant for more extensive evaluation of pulmonary vasculature function in DS patients so as to understand the precise incidence and etiology for this condition. PH significantly increases morbidity and mortality and if not identified and treated appropriately may have added detrimental effects on this population already at risk. Further studies examining the mechanism, possible genetic variations, and treatment for PH in this complicated population are needed to improve outcomes.

References

[1] Improved national prevalence estimates for 18 selected major birth defects--United States, 1999-2001. *MMWR Morb Mortal Wkly Rep* 2006;54:1301-5.

[2] Menendez M. Down syndrome, Alzheimer's disease and seizures. *Brain Dev* 2005;27:246-52.

[3] Matsuda Y, Sano N, Watanabe S, Oki S, Shibata T. Atlanto-occipital hypermobility in subjects with Down's syndrome. *Spine* 1995;20:2283-6.

[4] Unachak K, Tanpaiboon P, Pongprot Y, et al. Thyroid functions in children with Down's syndrome. *J Med Assoc Thai* 2008;91:56-61.

[5] Fonseca CT, Amaral DM, Ribeiro MG, Beserra IC, Guimaraes MM. Insulin resistance in adolescents with Down syndrome: a cross-sectional study. *BMC Endocr Disord* 2005;5:6.

[6] Freeman SB, Bean LH, Allen EG, et al. Ethnicity, sex, and the incidence of congenital heart defects: a report from the National Down Syndrome Project. *Genet Med* 2008;10:173-80.

[7] Aquino A, Domini M, Rossi C, Sardella L, Palka G, Chiesa PL. Correlation between Down's syndrome and malformations of pediatric surgical interest. *J Pediatr Surg* 1998;33:1380-2.

[8] Kallen B, Mastroiacovo P, Robert E. Major congenital malformations in Down syndrome. *Am J Med Genet* 1996;65:160-6.

[9] Vyas P, Roberts I. Down myeloid disorders: a paradigm for childhood preleukaemia and leukaemia and insights into normal megakaryopoiesis. *Early Hum Dev* 2006;82:767-73.

[10] Whitlock JA. Down syndrome and acute lymphoblastic leukaemia. *Br J Haematol* 2006;135:595-602.

[11] Rodriguez de al Nuez AL, Sanchez Dominguez T, Villa-Elizaga I, Subira ML. Down's syndrome and immune function. *Am J Dis Child* 1982;136:81.

[12] Ugazio AG, Maccario R, Notarangelo LD, Burgio GR. Immunology of Down syndrome: a review. *Am J Med Genet Suppl* 1990;7:204-12.

[13] Simonneau G, Galie N, Rubin LJ, et al. Clinical classification of pulmonary hypertension. *J Am Coll Cardiol* 2004;43:5S-12S.

[14] Rohde M, Banner J. Respiratory tract malacia: possible cause of sudden death in infancy and early childhood. *Acta Paediatr* 2006;95:867-70.

[15] Levine OR, Simpser M. Alveolar hypoventilation and cor pulmonale associated with chronic airway obstruction in infants with Down syndrome. *Clin Pediatr* (Phila) 1982;21:25-9.

[16] Marcus CL, Keens TG, Bautista DB, von Pechmann WS, Ward SL. Obstructive sleep apnea in children with Down syndrome. *Pediatrics* 1991;88:132-9.
[17] Lefaivre JF, Cohen SR, Burstein FD, et al. Down syndrome: identification and surgical management of obstructive sleep apnea. *Plast Reconstr Surg* 1997;99:629-37.
[18] Kasian GF, Duncan WJ, Tyrrell MJ, Oman-Ganes LA. Elective oro-tracheal intubation to diagnose sleep apnea syndrome in children with Down's syndrome and ventricular septal defect. *Can J Cardiol* 1987;3:2-5.
[19] Ayeni TI, Roper HP. Pulmonary hypertension resulting from upper airways obstruction in Down's syndrome. *J R Soc Med* 1998;91:321-2.
[20] Bloch K, Witztum A, Wieser HG, Schmid S, Russi E. [Obstructive sleep apnea syndrome in a child with trisomy 21]. *Monatsschr Kinderheilkd* 1990;138:817-22.
[21] Fernandez Pastor FJ, Paez Gonzalez R, Mateos Perez G, Benito Bernal AI, Gil Sanchez A. [Pulmonary hypertension in a patient with Down syndrome and chronic upper airway obstruction]. *An Pediatr* (Barc) 2005;62:178-9.
[22] Hoch B, Barth H. Cheyne-Stokes respiration as an additional risk factor for pulmonary hypertension in a boy with trisomy 21 and atrioventricular septal defect. *Pediatr Pulmonol* 2001;31:261-4.
[23] Rowland TW, Nordstrom LG, Bean MS, Burkhardt H. Chronic upper airway obstruction and pulmonary hypertension in Down's syndrome. *Am J Dis Child* 1981;135:1050-2.
[24] Hultcrantz E, Svanholm H. Down syndrome and sleep apnea--a therapeutic challenge. *Int J Pediatr Otorhinolaryngol* 1991;21:263-8.
[25] Clark RW, Schmidt HS, Schuller DE. Sleep-induced ventilatory dysfunction in Down's syndrome. *Arch Intern Med* 1980;140:45-50.
[26] Jacobs IN, Teague WG, Bland JW, Jr. Pulmonary vascular complications of chronic airway obstruction in children. *Arch Otolaryngol Head Neck Surg* 1997;123:700-4.
[27] Jacobs IN, Gray RF, Todd NW. Upper airway obstruction in children with Down syndrome. *Arch Otolaryngol Head Neck Surg* 1996;122:945-50.
[28] Wilson SK, Hutchins GM, Neill CA. Hypertensive pulmonary vascular disease in Down syndrome. *J Pediatr* 1979;95:722-6.
[29] Cooney TP, Thurlbeck WM. Pulmonary hypoplasia in Down's syndrome. *N Engl J Med* 1982;307:1170-3.

[30] Hasegawa N, Oshima M, Kawakami H, Hirano H. Changes in pulmonary tissue of patients with congenital heart disease and Down syndrome: a morphological and histochemical study. *Acta Paediatr Jpn* 1990;32:60-6.
[31] Galambos C. Alveolar Capillary Dysplasia in a Patient with Down's Syndrome. *Pediatr Dev Pathol* 2006;9:254-5; author reply 256.
[32] Shehata BM, Abramowsky CR. Alveolar capillary dysplasia in an infant with trisomy 21. *Pediatr Dev Pathol* 2005;8:696-700.
[33] Tibballs J, Chow CW. Incidence of alveolar capillary dysplasia in severe idiopathic persistent pulmonary hypertension of the newborn. *J Paediatr Child Health* 2002;38:397-400.
[34] Greenwood RD, Nadas AS. The clinical course of cardiac disease in Down's syndrome. *Pediatrics* 1976;58:893-7.
[35] Cantor WJ, Harrison DA, Moussadji JS, et al. Determinants of survival and length of survival in adults with Eisenmenger syndrome. *Am J Cardiol* 1999;84:677-81.
[36] Suzuki K, Yamaki S, Mimori S, et al. Pulmonary vascular disease in Down's syndrome with complete atrioventricular septal defect. *Am J Cardiol* 2000;86:434-7.
[37] Borowski A, Zeuchner M, Schickendantz S, Korb H. Efficacy of pulmonary artery banding in the prevention of pulmonary vascular obstructive disease. *Cardiology* 1994;85:207-15.
[38] Thieren M, Stijns-Cailteux M, Tremouroux-Wattiez M, et al. [Congenital heart diseases and obstructive pulmonary vascular diseases in Down's syndrome. Apropos of 142 children with trisomy 21]. *Arch Mal Coeur Vaiss* 1988;81:655-61.
[39] Calderon-Colmenero J, Flores A, Ramirez S, et al. [Surgical treatment results of congenital heart defects in children with Down's syndrome.]. *Arch Cardiol Mex* 2004;74:39-44.
[40] Kwiatkowska J, Tomaszewski M, Bielinska B, Potaz P, Erecinski J. Atrioventricular septal defect: clinical and diagnostic problems in children hospitalised in 1993-1998. *Med Sci Monit* 2000;6:1148-54.
[41] Chi TPLKJ. The pulmonary vascular bed in children with Down syndrome. *J Pediatr* 1975;86:533-8.
[42] Clapp S, Perry BL, Farooki ZQ, et al. Down's syndrome, complete atrioventricular canal, and pulmonary vascular obstructive disease. *J Thorac Cardiovasc Surg* 1990;100:115-21.

[43] Yamaki S, Horiuchi T, Sekino Y. Quantitative analysis of pulmonary vascular disease in simple cardiac anomalies with the Down syndrome. *Am J Cardiol* 1983;51:1502-6.
[44] Yamaki S, Yasui H, Kado H, et al. Pulmonary vascular disease and operative indications in complete atrioventricular canal defect in early infancy. *J Thorac Cardiovasc Surg* 1993;106:398-405.
[45] Ando H, Yasui H, Kado H, et al. [Total repair of complete atrioventricular canal: relationship between age at operation and late results]. *Nippon Kyobu Geka Gakkai Zasshi* 1989;37:265-73.
[46] Frid C, Thoren C, Book K, Bjork VO. Repair of complete atrioventricular canal. 15 year's experience. *Scand J Thorac Cardiovasc Surg* 1991;25:101-5.
[47] Okada H, Tsuboi H, Nishi K, et al. [Surgical treatment of ventricular septal defect associated with Down syndrome]. *Kyobu Geka* 1993;46:396-8.
[48] Lindberg L, Olsson AK, Jogi P, Jonmarker C. How common is severe pulmonary hypertension after pediatric cardiac surgery? *J Thorac Cardiovasc Surg* 2002;123:1155-63.
[49] Kawai T, Wada Y, Enmoto T, et al. Comparison of hemodynamic data before and after corrective surgery for Down's syndrome and ventricular septal defect. *Heart Vessels* 1995;10:154-7.
[50] Cua CL, Blankenship A, North AL, Hayes J, Nelin LD. Increased incidence of idiopathic persistent pulmonary hypertension in Down syndrome neonates. *Pediatr Cardiol* 2007;28:250-4.
[51] Southgate WM, Annibale DJ, Hulsey TC, Purohit DM. International experience with trisomy 21 infants placed on extracorporeal membrane oxygenation. *Pediatrics* 2001;107:549-52.
[52] Cannon BC, Feltes TF, Fraley JK, Grifka RG, Riddle EM, Kovalchin JP. Nitric oxide in the evaluation of congenital heart disease with pulmonary hypertension: factors related to nitric oxide response. *Pediatr Cardiol* 2005;26:565-9.
[53] Vazquez-Antona CA, Lomeli C, Buendia A, Vargas-Barron J. [Pulmonary hypertension in children with Down's syndrome and congenital heart disease. Is it really more severe?]. *Arch Cardiol Mex* 2006;76:16-27.
[54] Cappelli-Bigazzi M, Santoro G, Battaglia C, et al. Endothelial cell function in patients with Down's syndrome. *Am J Cardiol* 2004;94:392-5.
[55] Diller GP, van Eijl S, Okonko DO, et al. Circulating endothelial progenitor cells in patients with Eisenmenger syndrome and idiopathic pulmonary arterial hypertension. *Circulation* 2008;117:3020-30.

[56] Kageyama K, Hashimoto S, Nakajima Y, Shime N, Hashimoto S. The change of plasma endothelin-1 levels before and after surgery with or without Down syndrome. *Paediatr Anaesth* 2007;17:1071-7.

[57] Canter JA, Summar ML, Smith HB, et al. Genetic variation in the mitochondrial enzyme carbamyl-phosphate synthetase I predisposes children to increased pulmonary artery pressure following surgical repair of congenital heart defects: a validated genetic association study. *Mitochondrion* 2007;7:204-10.

[58] Cua CL, Cooke G, Taylor M, et al. Endothelial nitric oxide synthase polymorphisms associated with abnormal nitric oxide production are not over-represented in children with Down syndrome. *Congenit Heart Dis* 2006;1:169-74.

Index

A

abnormalities, 138, 139, 141
acetylcholine, 141
acid, 11, 39
acidosis, 126
acute, 142
adaptation, viii, 57
adenoidectomy, 139
adenopathy, 5
adenosine, 21, 22, 61
adenovirus, 34
administration, 141
adolescents, 142
adults, 38, 70, 72, 73, 74, 100, 116, 144
adventitia, 59
adverse effects, 23, 32, 124
adverse event, 28
age, 21, 64, 65, 66, 67, 68, 69, 74, 83, 102, 139, 140, 145
aggregation, 11
agonist, 31, 54
AIDS, 37
airways, 143
alkaline, 141
alkaline phosphatase, 141
alveoli, 139
American Heart Association, 98
amino, 112

amplitude, 17
anatomic levels, vii, 1, 5
androgen, 60
anemia, 33
angiogenesis, 40
anticoagulation, 22
antidepressant, 32
antinuclear antibodies, 7
antisense, 46
aorta, 105
apex, 19
apnea, 138, 143
apoptosis, 6, 7, 10, 13, 14, 17, 31, 32, 33, 34, 36, 37, 38, 41, 43, 54, 55, 56, 75
arrest, 102, 103, 105
arrhythmia, 64, 68, 88, 90
arterial blood gas, 82
arterial hypertension, vii, viii, 39, 40, 41, 42, 43, 44, 45, 46, 50, 53, 57, 58, 70, 71, 72, 73, 74, 81, 98, 99, 100, 131, 133, 134, 145
arterial wall, vii, 1, 5, 6, 33
arteries, 6, 45, 60, 76, 77
arterioles, ix, 15, 17, 59, 118, 119, 120, 122, 129
arteriosclerosis, 2
artery, ix, 5, 8, 10, 14, 15, 18, 31, 32, 33, 34, 39, 41, 43, 44, 47, 48, 50, 54, 55, 66, 67, 75, 81, 82, 85, 89, 90, 103, 104, 105, 106,

111, 115, 117, 118, 119, 127, 133, 140, 141, 144, 146
assessment, x, 36, 47, 61, 70, 81, 94, 95, 96, 118, 121, 125, 126, 129, 131
atrial septal defect, 10, 38, 72, 74, 80, 85, 89, 96, 100
atrium, 84, 88
atrophy, 114
autoantibodies, 7
autoimmune diseases, 10
autoimmune hepatitis, 120

B

bacterial infection, 112
beneficial effect, 30, 53
benefits, ix, 22, 58, 69
bioavailability, 37
biomarkers, 120
biomolecules, 60
biopsies, 139
biopsy, 61, 72, 95, 99
biosynthesis, 70
birth, 142
bleeding, 22
blood, viii, 2, 20, 33, 50, 57, 59, 64, 65, 71, 102, 105, 106, 109, 119, 120, 132, 139, 140, 141
blood flow, viii, 50, 57, 59, 64, 71, 119, 120, 132, 139, 140, 141
blood pressure, 2, 59, 105
blood transfusion, 109
body weight, 29
bone, viii, 5, 9, 30, 31, 36, 40, 53, 54, 57, 60, 120
bone marrow, 30, 53
Boston, 137
bradykinin, 15, 31, 45, 54
brain, 131
breakdown, 12
breathing, 4, 138
bronchitis, 2
bronchodilator, 32

bundle branch block, 17, 121

C

C reactive protein, 103
calcitonin, 112
calcium, viii, 2, 9, 12, 13, 14, 15, 21, 22, 30, 32, 48, 49, 50, 85, 123
calcium channel blocker, 21, 48, 49, 85, 123
calcium-channel blockers, viii, 2, 21, 22, 48, 50
cancer, 33, 53, 56
candidates, x, 61, 118, 122, 125, 131, 133, 134
capillary, 3, 4, 81, 83, 138, 139, 144
carbon, 39, 121
carbon dioxide, 121
carbon monoxide, 39
carcinogenesis, 6
cardiac arrest, 85
cardiac catheterization, 37, 61, 83, 94, 98
cardiac output, 19, 61, 80, 82, 104, 120, 121, 124, 125, 127, 128, 129
cardiac surgery, viii, 57, 58, 111, 112, 113, 116, 124, 140, 145
cardiomyopathy, ix, 117, 119, 121, 122, 124, 129, 131
cardiopulmonary, 140
cardiopulmonary bypass, 40, 80, 85, 102, 103, 114, 115
cardiotonic, 85
cardiovascular risk, 33
caspases, 32
catheter, 90, 95, 106, 123, 125
catheterizations, 82
CDC, 114
cell, 145
cell culture, 17
cell death, 34, 40, 55
cell lines, 33
central nervous system, 9
ceruloplasmin, 102, 107, 109
channel blocker, viii, 2, 21, 22, 48, 50

chemokines, 7
Cheyne-Stokes respiration, 143
childhood, 71, 81, 95, 142
children, vii, x, 39, 50, 60, 63, 66, 67, 68, 70, 71, 75, 81, 95, 98, 99, 137, 142, 143, 144, 145, 146
cholesterol, 15
chronic hypoxia, 9, 11, 12, 14, 40, 55
chronic obstructive pulmonary disease, 49, 138
chronic renal failure, 5
chronic thromboembolic pulmonary hypertension (CTEPH), ix, 102, 104
circulation, ix, 10, 54, 103, 104, 118, 119, 141
cirrhosis, ix, 117, 121, 130, 132, 134, 135
classes, 2, 27, 62
classification, 3, 35, 41, 60, 62, 71, 109, 138, 142
clinical presentation, 3, 121
clinical symptoms, ix, 118, 139
clinical syndrome, 35
closure, 61, 62, 64, 65, 66, 72, 74, 75, 80, 82, 86, 90, 94, 96, 100, 105
cohort, 139
collagen, 47, 59
combination therapy, viii, 2, 21, 28, 30, 35
communication, 74
compliance, 20, 66
complications, 36, 104, 112, 118, 119, 135, 143
compression, 5
congenital heart disease, 9, 17, 29, 60, 64, 70, 71, 72, 73, 74, 80, 94, 98, 99, 100, 139, 144, 145
Congenital heart disease (CHD), viii, 57
congenital malformations, 142
connective tissue, 7, 10, 59, 60
consensus, 21, 82
consumption, 111
contraceptives, 21
control group, 20
controlled studies, 22, 62

controlled trials, 24, 27, 28
controversial, 22
COPD, 4
cor pulmonale, 129, 142
coronary artery bypass graft, 114, 116
coronary bypass surgery, 116
correlation, 15, 18, 25, 102, 109, 141
correlations, 72
CPB, 80, 85, 102, 103, 105, 106, 109, 110, 111
cross-sectional, 142
cross-sectional study, 142
CRP, 102, 103, 106, 109
culture, 10, 75
cyanosis, viii, 29, 57, 58
cytokines, ix, 7, 13, 15, 102, 104, 109, 110, 111, 112, 113, 115, 116
Czech Republic, 101, 113, 116

D

damages, iv, 139
database, 82, 124, 134, 135, 140
death, 142
deaths, 88, 89, 102, 109, 139
defects, 45, 58, 70, 72, 74, 75, 83, 96, 98, 99, 139, 142, 144, 146
deficiencies, 11
degradation, 17
demographics, 140
depolarization, 9, 14, 32
deposition, 9
depression, 103
destruction, 9
detection, 48, 112
developed countries, 58
deviation, 17, 20
diabetes, 33
diagnostic criteria, 119
dialysis, 5
diastole, 20
diastolic pressure, 2
dilated cardiomyopathy, 15, 44

dilation, 18, 19, 121
direct action, 10
disease progression, 32
diseases, 3, 7, 18, 19, 33, 35, 71, 144
disorder, x, 137, 138
displacement, 47
distress, 114
distribution, 87
diuretic, 85, 123
dizziness, 17
donor, 141
dopamine, 26
doppler, 51
Down syndrome, x, 137, 138, 142, 143, 144, 145, 146
drug interaction, 28
drugs, 6, 62, 124
DS population, x, 137, 139, 141
dyspepsia, 26
dysplasia, 138, 139, 144
Dysplasia, 144
dyspnea, 17, 18, 21

E

echocardiogram, x, 118
edema, 26, 33, 104
Eisenmenger syndrome (ES), viii, 57, 58, 59
elafin, 47
elastase inhibitors, 34
elastin, 17, 41, 59
electrocardiogram, 121
ELISA, 106
emphysema, 2
encoding, 9, 34, 36
endothelial cells, 10, 12, 15, 27, 31, 36, 37, 38, 39, 45, 56, 59, 60
endothelial dysfunction, ix, 10, 33, 59, 60, 118, 120, 125, 129
endothelial progenitor cells, 145
endothelin-1, 146
endothelin-receptor antagonists, viii, 2, 21, 27

endothelium, 6, 7, 12, 14, 15, 16, 45, 59, 120, 124, 128, 141
enlargement, 18, 138
environment, 128
enzyme, 11, 28, 46, 80, 146
enzymes, 11, 123, 124
epidemiology, 37
estrogen, 120
ETA, 12, 27
etiology, ix, 118, 120, 129, 138, 141
Europe, 24, 27
evidence, x, 6, 23, 29, 40, 83, 98, 118
evolution, 37, 71, 112
excretion, 39
exercise, ix, 2, 23, 24, 27, 28, 48, 51, 52, 58, 63, 68, 82, 104, 132
exertion, 17, 22, 84, 88, 121
experimental condition, 128
exposure, 4
extracellular matrix, 6, 9, 17, 59

F

factorial, 138
family members, 82
fasudil, viii, 2, 14, 21, 30, 42, 43
fatty acids, 33
fibers, 19, 59
fibrillation, 84, 89
fibroblasts, 5, 13, 15, 59
fibrosis, vii, 1, 2, 5, 30, 53, 71, 120, 122
flow, 139, 140, 141
fluoxetine, 31
formation, 6
fractures, 33
free radicals, 37

G

gastrointestinal, 138
gene expression, 38, 40, 112, 114
gene therapy, 32
gene transfer, 14, 15, 38, 44, 55

general anesthesia, 85
general practitioner, 86
genes, 9, 12, 34, 36
genetic alteration, 60
genetic mutations, 6
genetic predisposition, 5, 9, 10, 14
genetics, 115
Germany, 105, 107
germline mutations, 36
ghrelin, viii, 2, 21, 31
glycogen, 5
glycoside, 85
grades, 61, 70
grading, 61
groups, 141
growth, 7, 8, 11, 12, 13, 16, 17, 26, 31, 34, 36, 40, 45, 55, 56, 59, 71, 120, 124
growth factor, 7, 8, 12, 13, 16, 17, 26, 34, 40, 45, 56, 59, 71, 124
growth hormone, 31
guidelines, 81, 95, 96, 98, 105, 122, 131

H

half-life, 112, 123
harmful effects, 112
headache, 123
health, 14, 51
heart, 139, 142, 144, 145, 146
Heart, 137, 145, 146
heart disease, viii, 3, 4, 57, 94, 139, 144, 145
heart failure, 17, 29, 33, 61, 74, 83, 84, 88, 89, 118, 130
heart murmur, 84, 86, 88
heme, 11, 38, 39
heme oxygenase, 38, 39
hemodialysis, 126
hemodynamic, 145
hemoglobin, 9, 25, 37, 86, 87, 93, 94
hemoglobinopathies, 3, 9
hemolytic anemia, 4
hemoptysis, 58, 86, 88, 90
hepatotoxicity, 26

hereditary hemorrhagic telangiectasia, 3, 9, 36
heterogeneity, 6, 96
heterozygote, 16
histochemical, 144
histology, 7
history, 49, 82, 100
HIV, 10, 37, 38, 40
HIV-1, 37, 38, 40
HO-1, 11, 130
homeostasis, 11, 141
hospital death, 83
human, 3, 7, 10, 12, 15, 32, 37, 40, 41, 44, 50, 54, 60, 81, 95
human development, 81, 95
human immunodeficiency virus, 3, 7, 10, 37, 60
human subjects, 12
hydrogen, 11, 39
hyperplasia, 15, 25, 44, 54, 55, 59, 60
hypertension, iv, vii, ix, x, 1, 2, 3, 4, 6, 7, 21, 25, 35, 44, 45, 47, 48, 49, 50, 51, 52, 61, 64, 66, 67, 70, 76, 80, 82, 99, 117, 118, 119, 129, 130, 131, 132, 133, 134, 135, 137, 138, 140, 142, 143, 144, 145
Hypertension, 137
hypertrophy, 17, 25, 27, 31, 59, 85, 86, 89, 118, 120
hypoplasia, 139, 143
hypotension, 111, 113, 124
hypothermia, 126
hypothesis, ix, 6, 7, 10, 102, 105, 122
hypoventilation, 138, 142
hypoxemia, 4, 22, 46, 121, 138
hypoxia, 4, 6, 9, 11, 13, 36, 38, 42, 55, 68, 126

I

ideal, 95
identification, vii, 1, 9, 143
idiopathic, viii, 7, 9, 12, 16, 39, 41, 43, 44, 45, 48, 49, 51, 52, 53, 57, 60, 141, 144, 145

idiopathic pulmonary hypertension, 39, 44, 48, 49, 51, 52, 53, 60
IL-8, ix, 102, 103, 104, 105, 106, 109, 110, 111, 113
imatinib, viii, 2, 21, 30, 53, 134
immune function, 142
immune system, 104
immunodeficiency, 3
immunoreactivity, 46
improvements, 31, 63, 109
in vitro, 39, 44, 45, 112
in vivo, 44, 45, 113
incidence, 30, 63, 64, 95, 138, 139, 140, 141, 142, 145
increased workload, 118
independent variable, 87
individuals, 18, 64, 138, 141
induction, 31
infancy, 81, 95, 142, 145
infants, 68, 98, 139, 142, 145
infarction, 38
infection, 7, 10, 21, 37, 88, 90, 104, 105, 113, 115, 123
inflammation, vii, 1, 5, 6, 11, 15, 112, 115, 116
inflammatory cells, 6, 59
influenza, 21
informed consent, 82, 97, 105
inhibition, 10, 30, 37, 42, 43, 53, 54, 75
inhibitor, 11, 14, 26, 27, 31, 34, 42, 43, 47, 52, 53, 73, 123, 124
initiation, 14, 20, 123, 128
injury, iv, 7, 10, 13, 56, 111, 112, 114, 128
insulin, 13, 33, 40
insulin sensitivity, 33
integrin, 17
integrins, 34
intensive care unit, 108, 134
interdependence, 131, 132
interference, 106
interleukin-8, 103
internalization, 43, 54
intervention, vii, 1, 70

intra-aortic balloon pump, 128
intravenously, 106, 123
intrinsic, 138, 141
ischemia, 126, 128
issues, x, 63, 137, 138
Italy, 3

K

K^+, 43, 44, 54
kinase activity, 13
kinetics, 111, 113

L

LA, 143
laminar, 10
lead, 7, 9, 12, 15, 110, 139
left ventricle, 19, 74, 86
leptin, 114
lesions, 7, 12, 15, 16, 27, 31, 36, 37, 38, 40, 59, 60, 64, 76, 81, 95, 120, 138, 139, 140
leukemia, 30, 142
leukotrienes, 15
LH, 142
liberation, 112
life expectancy, 119
life quality, 80, 97
ligand, 33, 56
links, 138
liver, vii, ix, 22, 28, 117, 118, 119, 120, 121, 122, 123, 124, 125, 126, 127, 128, 129, 130, 131, 132, 133, 134, 135
liver cirrhosis, ix, 117, 118, 120, 121
liver disease, x, 22, 118, 119, 121, 131, 135
liver transplant, vii, ix, 117, 118, 119, 120, 121, 122, 123, 124, 125, 126, 127, 128, 129, 130, 131, 132, 133, 134, 135
local anesthesia, 82
lumen, 140
lung, 138, 139, 140, 141
lung disease, 4, 138
lupus, 10

Index 153

lymphocytes, 7

M

macroglossia, 138
macrophages, 7
magnetic resonance, 19, 48
magnetic resonance imaging, 19, 48
magnitude, ix, 58
maintenance, 141
majority, ix, 117, 139
management, 47, 49, 50, 58, 69, 70, 75, 81, 95, 96, 98, 100, 104, 111, 114, 115, 122, 126, 130, 131, 133, 143
mass, 19, 20
matrix, 6, 7, 17, 34, 46, 52
matrix metalloproteinase, 6, 17, 34, 46
MBP, 68
mean arterial pressure, 106, 111
measurements, 17, 18, 19, 20, 21
mechanical ventilation, 126
median, 68, 102, 105, 107
medical, x, 58, 67, 73, 82, 83, 86, 96, 137, 138, 139
medication, 23, 24, 69
meta-analysis, 22
Metabolic, 5
metabolites, 11, 33, 39
methylation, 60
mice, 12, 13, 15, 37, 38, 40, 41, 42, 44, 45, 47, 56
migration, 6, 9, 14, 17, 30, 33, 42
mitochondrial, 146
mitogen, 12, 32
mitogens, 10
mitral stenosis, 41
mitral valve, 133
MMP, 17
models, 11, 13, 14, 15, 17, 33, 47
molecules, ix, 6, 11, 13, 15, 40, 118, 120
monocyte chemoattractant protein, 45
morbidity, vii, 1, 2, 21, 63, 141

morphogenetic protein receptor, viii, 5, 9, 31, 57, 60
morphological, 144
morphology, 19, 61, 99
morphometric, 62, 72
mortality, vii, 1, 2, 21, 29, 48, 63, 67, 68, 69, 82, 87, 88, 90, 102, 104, 116, 125, 141
mortality rate, 68
mortality risk, 29
Moses, 45
MRI, 48
muscle mass, 20
Mustard operation, viii, 58, 76, 77
mutation, 6, 36
mutations, viii, 9, 17, 57, 60, 71
myelofibrosis, 30
myeloid, 142
myeloproliferative disorders, 3, 5, 30, 53
myocardium, 19
myofibroblasts, 6, 7, 59
myosin, 13

N

nares, 83
nausea, 123
nebulizer, 124, 128
necrosis, 103
neonatal, 138, 140
neonates, 46, 145
Ni, 145
nitrates, 26
nitric oxide, 9, 14, 22, 24, 27, 31, 33, 37, 38, 40, 42, 48, 49, 50, 56, 59, 61, 65, 69, 72, 74, 81, 83, 98, 99, 112, 114, 120, 122, 124, 127, 128, 133, 141, 145, 146
nitric oxide (NO), 141
nitric oxide synthase, 33, 42, 112, 114, 146
nitrite, 115
non-surgical therapy, 91, 92, 96
norepinephrine, 102, 106, 109, 110, 111
normal, 140, 142
normal distribution, 87

null, 11, 12, 15, 38

O

obesity, 13, 139
observations, 139, 141
obstruction, vii, 1, 2, 4, 5, 68, 83, 100, 102, 109, 119, 138, 142, 143
obstructive sleep apnea, 143
occlusion, 62, 65, 95, 100, 119
Oman, 143
one-way flap, viii, 58
open heart surgery, 113
open lung biopsy, 100
optimization, 129
organ, 75, 104, 115
organize, 15
orthopnea, 121
outpatients, 50
overproduction, 112
oxidative stress, 11, 56
oxide, 145, 146
oxygen, 10, 22, 43, 55, 61, 63, 68, 69, 83, 86, 94, 96, 138, 141
oxygen saturation, 138
oxygenation, 140, 145
oxyhemoglobin, 10

P

pain, x, 17, 23, 24, 26, 118, 123
palliative, 58, 63, 64, 66, 67, 68, 69, 70, 76
palpitations, x, 118
parenchyma, 18, 111, 139
parenchymal, 139
patent ductus arteriosus, 10, 64, 65, 70, 72, 100
pathogenesis, iv, vii, 1, 2, 5, 9, 14, 15, 17, 32, 34, 37, 56, 59, 111
pathology, 70, 122
pathophysiological, 2, 3
pathophysiology, viii, 6, 35, 57, 58, 60, 130, 131

pathways, vii, 1, 7, 11, 13, 15
patients, 138, 139, 140, 141, 144, 145
PCR, 60, 96
PCT, 102, 103, 104, 106, 107, 109, 110, 111, 112, 113
pediatric, 138, 142, 145
peptide, 16, 31, 32, 34, 40, 54, 121, 131
percentile, 84, 88
perfusion, 24, 40, 126
permission, iv, 127
persistent pulmonary hypertension of the newborn, 140, 144
persistent pulmonary hypertension of the newborn (PPHN), 140
pharmacokinetics, 28
Philadelphia, 114
phosphate, 11, 33, 146
phosphodiesterase type 5 inhibitors, 2, 21
physical exercise, 21
physicians, 82, 85
physiology, vii, 65, 73, 141
pilot study, 24, 28, 32, 48, 105
pioglitazone, 33
placebo, 24, 25, 28, 49, 51, 63, 73, 132
plasma levels, 41, 109, 112, 114, 146
plasma membrane, 15
platelet activating factor, 8
platelet aggregation, 12
platelets, 6, 7, 11
polycythemia, 68
polymorphisms, 14, 131, 146
polysomnography, 139
population, x, 10, 81, 83, 87, 95, 137, 138, 141
portal hypertension, ix, 9, 117, 118, 119, 120, 121, 129, 130
portal vein, 123, 132
positive correlation, 111
potassium, 9, 13, 14, 32, 36, 43, 44, 55, 59
PPHN, 140
pressure gradient, 81, 132
prevention, 34, 144

Index

primary pulmonary hypertension, 2, 36, 40, 43, 46, 47, 48, 49, 50, 51, 52, 54, 60, 72, 75, 95, 99, 120, 124, 134
probability, 86
production, 141, 146
progenitor cells, 141, 145
prognosis, 2, 19, 27, 29, 97, 104
pro-inflammatory, 15, 59, 111, 112
proliferation, vii, viii, 1, 2, 5, 6, 9, 10, 11, 12, 13, 14, 15, 16, 17, 25, 27, 30, 31, 32, 33, 36, 38, 40, 43, 46, 57, 59, 60, 71, 120, 140
prostacyclin, viii, 2, 11, 21, 22, 23, 24, 27, 31, 39, 49, 50, 59, 65, 70, 73, 75, 99, 120, 123, 132
prosthesis, 74
protection, 44
protective role, 13
protein kinase C, 12, 42, 43
proteinase, 46
proteins, 7, 10, 37, 103, 106, 109, 113
pulmonary arterial hypertension (PAH), viii, 57, 58
pulmonary arteries, 4, 6, 9, 12, 17, 25, 35, 41, 54, 59, 67, 70, 72, 75
pulmonary artery pressure, ix, 2, 54, 65, 66, 68, 80, 81, 82, 83, 85, 89, 103, 104, 106, 108, 117, 119, 127, 133, 140, 141, 146
pulmonary circulation, viii, 5, 10, 12, 21, 33, 38, 58, 59, 60, 61, 62, 64, 119, 120
pulmonary edema, 23
pulmonary embolism, 2, 4
Pulmonary endarterectomy (PEA), ix, 102, 104
pulmonary hypertension, vii, ix, x, 1, 2, 3, 4, 7, 16, 17, 25, 26, 32, 34, 35, 36, 37, 38, 39, 40, 41, 42, 43, 44, 45, 46, 47, 48, 49, 50, 51, 52, 53, 54, 55, 56, 59, 60, 61, 62, 64, 65, 66, 67, 70, 71, 72, 74, 75, 76, 77, 79, 80, 82, 94, 95, 96, 98, 99, 100, 102, 103, 104, 114, 115, 116, 117, 118, 119, 120, 121, 122, 123, 124, 128, 130, 131, 132, 133, 134, 137, 138, 140, 142, 143, 144, 145

pulmonary vascular resistance, vii, viii, ix, 1, 2, 6, 12, 58, 62, 63, 66, 74, 75, 79, 81, 85, 89, 98, 99, 100, 104, 117, 118, 131
pulmonary vascular resistance (PVR), ix, 2, 79, 81, 104, 118

Q

quality of life, 51

R

RANTES, 7, 15, 45
reactants, ix, 102, 105
reactive oxygen, 9
reactivity, 46, 61, 94, 122, 132
receptors, 12, 27, 34, 40, 43, 44, 46, 54, 71, 123
recognition, 36, 141
recommendations, iv
reconstruction, 35
regression, 14, 34, 46, 61, 75, 86, 87, 93, 94
regression analysis, 86, 87
regression equation, 87
regression model, 87
relationship, 145
relaxation, 27
reliability, 95
relief, 60
remodeling, vii, viii, 1, 2, 5, 6, 7, 8, 9, 12, 13, 14, 15, 16, 17, 20, 23, 30, 33, 35, 41, 43, 48, 55, 57, 58, 59, 62, 64, 66, 69, 115, 124
remodelling, 36, 71
repair, viii, 29, 58, 59, 62, 63, 67, 69, 70, 72, 74, 75, 76, 83, 94, 140, 145, 146
repression, 10, 34
resistance, ix, 2, 58, 61, 63, 64, 69, 95, 96, 103, 108, 118, 119, 121, 124, 125, 128, 140, 141, 142
resolution, 140
respiration, 143
respiratory problems, 138

response, 2, 6, 10, 11, 12, 13, 14, 16, 17, 20, 21, 22, 25, 30, 32, 48, 49, 50, 61, 94, 103, 104, 110, 111, 112, 113, 114, 115, 125, 141, 145
restoration, 48
rheumatoid arthritis, 10
rhythm, 86
right atrium, 93
right ventricle, 19, 35, 41, 48, 54, 118
risk, x, 2, 14, 22, 32, 37, 55, 61, 63, 66, 83, 94, 95, 96, 104, 120, 121, 122, 123, 124, 125, 128, 130, 131, 137, 138, 139, 140, 141, 143
risk factors, 14, 83, 94, 120, 130, 131, 139, 140
rodents, 15, 44
rosiglitazone, 56

S

safety, 25, 28, 32, 49, 52, 56, 63
sarcoidosis, 5
saturation, ix, 58, 63, 67, 68, 96
Schmid, 143
scleroderma, 22, 37
scope, 95
secrete, 15
secretion, 37, 141
seizures, 142
sensing, 43, 55
sensitivity, 121
sensitization, 30
sepsis, 111, 112, 113
septum, 20
serine, 17, 46, 47
serotonin, 8, 9, 14, 15, 17, 32, 42, 44, 47, 59
serum, 12, 32, 110, 112, 113, 115, 116
severity, 138, 140, 141
sex, 86, 120, 139, 142
shape, 15
shear, viii, 6, 10, 38, 58, 59, 62
sheep, 45
shortness of breath, x, 26, 118

shunts, 138
sickle cell, 9, 36, 37
side effects, 123
signaling pathway, 31
significance level, 107
signs, 17, 19, 21, 22, 111, 126
simvastatin, viii, 2, 14, 21, 31
sinus rhythm, 126
skeletal muscle, 114
sleep, 138, 139, 143
smooth muscle, 5, 6, 8, 9, 10, 11, 12, 13, 14, 15, 17, 25, 27, 30, 31, 32, 33, 36, 39, 40, 42, 43, 44, 46, 49, 50, 54, 55, 56, 59, 60, 75, 112, 114
smooth muscle cells, 9, 10, 12, 13, 14, 15, 17, 27, 30, 32, 33, 39, 40, 42, 43, 44, 49, 50, 54, 59, 112, 114
sodium, 50, 73
species, 9
speculation, 140
spinal anesthesia, 134
splenomegaly, 123, 132
standard deviation, 86, 108
state, ix, 14, 15, 22, 94, 117, 118, 120, 134
stenosis, 83, 138
stimulus, 6, 113
strategy use, 64
stratification, 95
stress, viii, ix, 6, 10, 38, 58, 59, 62, 114, 118, 120, 125
stroke, 64
stroma, 7
structural changes, 70, 72
structure, 48, 72
subgroups, 134, 135
Sun, 42, 56, 75
superior vena cava, 105
suppression, 46, 75
surface area, 80, 83
surfactant, 141
surgery, 139, 140, 141, 145, 146
surgical, 139, 142, 143, 146
surgical intervention, 104

Index

survival, viii, ix, 12, 13, 19, 23, 29, 37, 47, 49, 50, 56, 57, 68, 69, 72, 79, 80, 81, 86, 90, 91, 92, 96, 99, 104, 119, 124, 129, 134, 140, 144
survival rate, 19, 68, 96, 104
Swan-Ganz catheter, 106
symptoms, viii, x, 2, 21, 23, 24, 25, 26, 34, 58, 62, 104, 118, 121, 123, 139
syndrome, viii, x, 25, 29, 37, 51, 53, 57, 58, 59, 67, 69, 70, 71, 72, 73, 74, 83, 100, 103, 104, 112, 114, 115, 120, 130, 134, 135, 137, 138, 142, 143, 144, 145, 146
synergistic effect, 69
synthesis, 11, 15
systemic circulation, 141
systemic sclerosis, 10, 37
systolic pressure, x, 18, 20, 118, 121

T

T cell, 10
Taiwan, 57
target, 13, 41, 56
techniques, 19
telangiectasia, 36
telephone, 86
tension, viii, 2, 120
testing, 22, 61, 94, 107
TGA, 64, 67, 68, 69
TGF, 8, 9, 36, 59, 71
Thai, 142
therapeutic approaches, 69
therapeutics, 56
therapy, x, 12, 14, 22, 23, 24, 25, 26, 32, 38, 39, 41, 49, 50, 51, 52, 58, 66, 69, 72, 73, 74, 75, 80, 91, 92, 95, 96, 99, 118, 119, 120, 123, 125, 126, 128, 129, 132, 133
thiazolidinediones, 33
thrombocytopenia, 123
thrombocytosis, 9
thrombomodulin, 120
thrombosis, vii, 1, 5, 6, 11, 16, 22, 25, 49, 129
thyroid, 3, 5, 112

thyroid gland, 112
time, 138, 139, 141
TIMP, 17
tissue, 3, 12, 15, 17, 32, 59, 60, 72, 112, 115, 139, 141, 144
TNF, 32, 37
tonsillectomy, 139
toxic effect, ix, 118
trachea, 138
tracheostomy, 139
trafficking, 15
traits, 7
transcatheter, 62
transcription, 10, 13, 33, 40, 43
transcription factors, 33
transduction, 10, 45
transforming growth factor, 9, 15, 59
transition, 140
translocation, 42
transplant, x, 118, 119, 120, 122, 125, 126, 129
transplantation, x, 25, 29, 63, 95, 104, 118, 119, 121, 122, 124, 125, 128, 129, 130, 134
transthoracic echocardiography, 121
trauma, 104, 111
treatment, vii, ix, 2, 3, 12, 18, 20, 21, 22, 24, 27, 28, 29, 30, 31, 35, 36, 38, 39, 40, 42, 49, 50, 51, 53, 54, 56, 58, 62, 63, 64, 65, 67, 68, 69, 73, 74, 75, 76, 79, 81, 82, 97, 102, 104, 113, 115, 123, 124, 125, 126, 128, 132, 133, 134, 135, 141, 144, 145
trial, 24, 25, 27, 28, 32, 49, 50, 63, 73, 96, 97, 109, 122, 132, 133
tricuspid valve, 66
triggers, 11, 13
trisomy, 138, 143, 144, 145
trisomy 21, 143, 144, 145
tumor, ix, 4, 5, 15, 45, 102, 104
tumor necrosis factor, ix, 102, 104
turnover, 54, 59
type 2 diabetes, 33, 56
tyrosine, 12

U

UK, 101, 106
United States, 142
upper airways, 143
urine, 12
USA, 3, 107

V

vagus nerve, 113
valve, 19, 66, 75, 81, 83
variables, 27, 86, 87, 95, 102, 107, 109
variation, 146
variations, 43, 141
vascular disease, 3. 45, 143, 144, 145
vascular effectors, vii, 1, 5, 11, 14, 16, 17
vascular proliferation/fibrosis, vii, 1, 2, 5
vascular wall, 13, 33, 120
vasculature, 10, 11, 12, 15, 33, 60, 66, 67, 94, 122, 123, 128, 139, 140, 141
vasoactive intestinal peptide, viii, 2, 12, 21, 40, 54
vasoconstriction, vii, 1, 5, 8, 9, 11, 12, 13, 14, 16, 27, 30, 32, 33, 36, 39, 42, 43, 44, 55, 59, 120, 123, 128
vasoconstrictor, 141
vasodilatation, 141
vasodilation, 25, 116, 141
vasodilator, viii, x, 11, 12, 21, 22, 23, 24, 25, 32, 42, 43, 50, 51, 57, 58, 61, 66, 69, 95, 98, 99, 113, 118, 119, 120, 122, 123, 124, 125, 126, 128, 129
vasopressor, 111
VEGF expression, 12
velocity, ix, 18, 20, 93, 118, 121
ventilation, 40, 88, 89, 105, 111, 138
ventricle, 118
ventricular septal defect, 10, 58, 70, 72, 75, 76, 77, 81, 85, 89, 93, 95, 97, 98, 99, 100, 139, 143, 145
ventricular septum, 61
vessel obstruction, vii, 1, 2, 5
vessels, 5, 9, 15, 59, 60
viral infection, 9
virus infection, 3
visualization, 19
vomiting, 26
VSD, 10, 58, 61, 64, 66, 67, 68, 69, 81, 85, 89, 96, 139, 140

W

weakness, 121
WHO, 2, 138
wild type, 11
windows, 80, 85, 89
withdrawal, 23
workload, 122